OXFORD MEDICAL PUBLICATIONS

THYROID DISEASE

the**facts**

the**facts**
THE FACTS FROM OXFORD UNIVERSITY PRESS

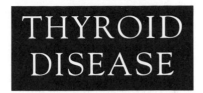

the**facts**

Third Edition

R. I. S. BAYLISS, KCVO, MD, FRCP

Consultant Endocrinologist,
Lister Hospital, London

and

W. M. G. TUNBRIDGE, MD, FRCP

Director of Postgraduate Medical Education and Training,
University of Oxford
Honorary Consultant Physician and Endocrinologist,
Radcliffe Infirmary, Oxford

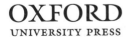

UNIVERSITY PRESS

OXFORD

UNIVERSITY PRESS

Great Clarendon Street, Oxford OX2 6DP

Oxford University Press is a department of the University of Oxford.
It furthers the University's objective of excellence in research, scholarship,
and education by publishing worldwide in

Oxford New York

Athens Auckland Bangkok Bogotá Buenos Aires Calcutta
Cape Town Chennai Dar es Salaam Delhi Florence Hong Kong Istanbul
Karachi Kuala Lumpur Madrid Melbourne Mexico City Mumbai
Nairobi Paris São Paulo Singapore Taipei Tokyo Toronto Warsaw

with associated companies in Berlin Ibadan

Oxford is a registered trade mark of Oxford University Press
in the UK and in certain other countries

Published in the United States
by Oxford University Press Inc., New York

© R.I. S. Bayliss and W. M. Tunbridge, 1998

The moral rights of the author have been asserted
Database right Oxford University Press (maker)

First edition published 1982
Second edition, 1991
Third edition, 1998
Reprinted 2000

A catalogue record for this book is available from the British Library

Library of Congress Cataloging in Publication Data
Bayliss, R. I. S. (Richard Ian Samuel)
Thyroid disease : the facts / R. I. S. Bayliss and W. M. G. Tunbridge—3rd ed.
(Oxford medical publications) (The facts)
Includes index.
1. Thyroid gland—Diseases—Popular works. I. Tunbridge, W. M. G.
(W. Michael G.) II. Title. III. Series. IV Series: The facts
(Oxford, England)
[DNLM: 1. Thyroid Diseases popular works. WK 200 B358t 1998]
RC655.B39 1998 616.4'4—dc21 98-3834

ISBN 0 19 262946 8 (Pbk)

Printed in Great Britain
on acid-free paper by
Biddles Ltd., Guildford & King's Lynn

Preface to third edition

For several reasons we have written this third edition of *Thyroid disease: the facts*. First, because thyroid disorders are common; secondly, because a proper understanding of their disease usually leads to a happier, less worrying outcome for the patient; thirdly, because progress in our understanding of thyroid diseases has grown since the second edition; and fourthly, because there has been continuing demand for the book. As in the past we have done our utmost to make it reader-friendly.

How common are thyroid disorders?

The prevalence of thyroid trouble varies considerably in different parts of the world and the incidence is always higher in females than in males. According to the World Health Organization, 200 million people world-wide have enlargement of their thyroid gland. Most of these goitres—and 'goitre' simply means enlargement of the thyroid gland—occur in people who live in parts of the world where there is lack of iodine in the diet, and later we shall see why iodine is so important. However, even in non-iodine-deficient areas, enlargement of the thyroid gland, so that it becomes visible, occurs in about 7 per cent of the population and is about ten times more common in women than men. In the United Kingdom some degree of underactivity of the thyroid gland affects about 10 per cent of all women over the age of 45 years. In the United States it is calculated that 10 million people have thyroid glands that are either overactive or underactive and in a significant proportion, perhaps as many as 2 million, this goes unrecognized for many months or years.

Why should you know about your condition?

Experience has taught us that the more people know about
their illness, the fewer are their fears. The greater their understanding of what is wrong, the better is their acceptance of,
and their co-operation with, the treatment and the more
they are able to help their doctor to help them.

This is certainly the case in people with disorders of the
thyroid gland, who benefit greatly from an understanding
of their disease. Notice that in this context we say 'people'
rather than 'patients' because many, despite requiring
treatment over many years and sometimes indefinitely,
may never actually feel ill.

Thus we write mainly for people who have some recognized disorder of the thyroid gland. We write also for their
relatives because many thyroid problems or related diseases
tend to run in families. If you have a parent, a sister or
brother, an aunt or uncle, or a cousin with thyroid disease,
you yourself are more likely to develop some thyroid disorder sooner or later. Self-diagnosis is not recommended
but, if you are aware of the possibility that you are vulner-
able and at risk, the sooner will you seek medical help if you
develop any of the symptoms or signs of the diseases
described in this book. However, in some instances, disorders of the thyroid gland are insidious in their onset and
the changes that occur are so slow to develop that you, and
those closest to you, may not be aware of them.

How the thyroid gland works, how it manufactures
hormones and how it is controlled are not hard to understand. We have tried to resist the temptation of being too
technical, but equally we have done our best not to sacrifice
scientific accuracy to over-simplification. In this third
edition, the glossary of terms at the end of the book has
been enlarged so that people have access to a fuller explana-
tion of medical and scientific words or concepts.

Today we live in an era of 'evidence-based medicine', by
which is meant that what advice a doctor gives or what

medication is prescribed should have been validated in scientifically controlled studies and trials. Based on such evidence a number of best practice protocols have been evolved for specific thyroid diseases by authoritative bodies. Increased adherence to these protocols by members of the medical profession at large will no doubt improve the standards of patient care. But medicine is not an exact science and probably never will be because no two people are exactly the same. People's susceptibility and their biological and psychological reactions to the same disease will always differ. Equally, doctors are likely to vary somewhat in their management of a patient's illness. No one course of action or method of treatment is always more 'right' than another.

You, or your relatives or friends, should not therefore be concerned that the treatment prescribed for you may not always follow exactly the practices advocated in this book. Apparent differences should not upset you because the fundamental scientific principles are widely accepted and likely to be much the same everywhere. Nevertheless, the precise details of management may vary from one patient to another, from one centre to another, and from one country to another, depending upon differences in the population being treated, the availability of technical facilities, laboratory expertise, and, in some instances, financial considerations. The art of embracing the special personal needs and wishes, the environmental or social factors, and the age, occupation, any concomitant disease(s), the severity of the condition, and the idiosyncrasies of an individual person with a thyroid disorder may contribute as much to the successful outcome as does the science.

In many countries lay support-groups for people with thyroid diseases have been established and proved a great help, at small cost, to many. These are listed in a glossary at the end of the book.

This book owes much to our colleagues in this country and abroad, not least in the United States. It is, however, the people from many lands, whom we have treated or supervised, who have undoubtedly taught us the most. To them go our special thanks.

We are grateful to Mr Keith Duguid, formerly Head of the Department of Medical Illustration at the Westminster Hospital, London, for the photographic work, and to Dr C. R. Bayliss, Consultant Radiologist at the Royal Devon and Exeter Hospital, for the illustrations used in Figures 4 to 7. Dr Robert Phillips, Consultant Radiotherapist and Oncologist at the Chelsea and Westminster Hospital kindly gave advice on the use of radioactive isotopes.

Finally, a word to the person who, having recently been diagnosed as having some thyroid disorder, is reading this book for the first time. We suggest you start by reading the chapter relevant to your condition. For example, if you have an overactive thyroid gland due to Graves' disease, read Chapters 4 and 5, or if you have an underactive gland due to Hashimoto's autoimmune thyroiditis, first read Chapters 7 and 8. Then go back to the beginning of the book and read Chapters 1 and 2. These will help to orientate you. Then read Chapter 3 about the tests and the investigations that have been, or will be, done to confirm the diagnosis of your illness. We hope this book will help you understand your condition.

London   R.I.S.B.
Oxford   W.M.G.T.
1998

the**facts**

CONTENTS

At the end of each chapter are answers to some of the more common questions that are asked by people about their thyroid disorder.

Contents

1
The thyroid gland

Where is the thyroid gland?

Normally the thyroid gland lies in the front of your neck just below your Adam's apple in the position where the knot of a man's tie would be (Fig. 1). The gland is H-shaped, like a butterfly, and consists of two lobes joined together in the middle. The left and right lobes, each about the size and shape of half a plum cut vertically, lie on either side of the mid-line against the windpipe, and are connected by a bridge of thyroid tissue, known as the isthmus, which runs across the front of the windpipe (Fig. 1).

In men a normal thyroid gland is seldom sufficiently large to be visible but in a young woman with a thin neck it may just be discernible, particularly when the chin is lifted up. If visible, the gland will be seen to move up and down as you swallow. In young people with a thin neck your doctor may be able to feel the two lobes of the thyroid but in older people with a short or thick neck it may not be palpable. A healthy gland is smooth and is not tender. It is not lumpy or hard.

In some perfectly normal people the gland may extend downwards to lie wholly or partially behind the upper part of the breast-bone or sternum. This is called a retrosternal thyroid.

Where does the thyroid come from?

In the baby developing in the womb (the fetus) the thyroid gland has its origins at the root of the tongue. As the fetus

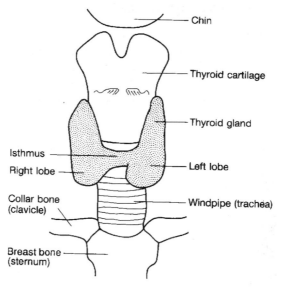

Figure 1 The anatomy of the thyroid gland.

grows, the thyroid moves down the neck and long before the baby is born it occupies the usual adult position. The path of this descent is marked by a narrow cord, the thyroglossal duct, running from the tongue (the glossus) to the neck. The bottom inch or two of this duct may contain thyroid tissue and is then called the pyramidal lobe. This extra lobe of the thyroid extends upwards from the isthmus and may lie in the mid-line or on one side of the larynx.

What happens if the thyroid does not descend properly?

Very rarely in some babies the thyroid gland does not descend properly and remains in its original position near the root of the tongue. A misplaced thyroid gland like this seldom functions properly, and is an important but uncommon cause of deficient thyroid hormone production in a new-born baby (Chapter 8).

What does the thyroid do?

The thyroid manufactures certain chemical substances (hormones) that are passed into the bloodstream and act on cells and tissues elsewhere in your body. Other glands, like the thyroid, that produce hormones, include the pituitary, the ovary and the testis, among others, and are known as endocrine glands.

The thyroid makes two hormones. One is thyroxine which, because it contains four atoms of iodine, is also called T_4. The other is triiodothyronine, which contains three iodine atoms, and for brevity is called T_3. Both these hormones are secreted into the bloodstream and carried round the body. In the distant tissues the thyroxine is converted to triiodothyronine and it is the triiodothyronine that actually influences the distant cells.

What do the thyroid hormones do?

The thyroid hormones control the speed of activity of all body cells. Too little of the thyroid hormones means that the body cells work at too slow a rate; too much causes them to work too fast.

Although the two thyroid hormones have a similar effect and influence the proper working of all body cells, their action is particularly evident in certain tissues and for certain functions. For example, the growth and development, both physical and mental, of a baby depend upon the presence of the correct amount of the thyroid hormones. We see this in the animal world too. Without thyroxine a tadpole will not change into a frog, and without thyroxine in the correct amount a new-born baby will not grow properly nor will his or her brain develop properly. Similarly, in a child too little thyroid hormone will slow up growth, whereas too much may make the child grow faster than normal. Thyroid hormones have a very noticeable effect, as we shall see later, on the heart and on the heart rate in particular.

Fundamentally, the thyroid hormones regulate the rate of oxygen consumption, which is another way of saying they control the speed of activity of the body cells. This metabolic action influences the utilization of the main components in our food—sugars, proteins, and fats. When there is thyroid deficiency, for example, the level of a particular fat, cholesterol, usually increases in the bloodstream. If this is allowed to continue, the arteries may become furred up because the cholesterol is deposited in the inner wall of the blood vessels, which become narrowed.

The manufacture of thyroid hormones

Thyroxine and triiodothyronine are formed in the cells of the thyroid gland. Both hormones contain iodine, which is essential for their manufacture or synthesis. This essential element is extracted from the bloodstream by the specialized thyroid cells. Inside the cells of the thyroid gland, the iodine is amalgamated with other substances in a number of chemical steps to form T_4 and T_3. Once formed, the two hormones are stored in 'parking areas' within the gland. The 'parked' hormones are released from storage into the bloodstream as and when the body cells need them.

Where does the iodine come from?

Normally iodine is provided by the food we eat, particularly fish. Iodine also comes from the soil, in which our crops grow to provide us with bread and vegetables, and on which cows graze to give us milk. The iodine is derived from the rain that falls on the soil, and this in turn comes from the water vapourized from the sea to form rain. In parts of the world far removed from the sea the soil is likely to be deficient in iodine. This happens in the land round the Congo in Central Africa, in the Andes in South America, the Himalayas in the Indian subcontinent, Switzerland in Central Europe, around the Great Lakes in the USA and in certain areas in other land masses such as Spain and Iran. People living in these areas may have difficulty in making thyroid hormones because there is insufficient iodine in their diet. Hence public-health measures have to be taken to supplement their dietary intake of iodine.

How is the secretion of thyroid hormones controlled?

What determines the amount of thyroid hormones secreted into the bloodstream? There is a clever mechanism for this which is simple to understand. Fundamentally it works like the control of the central heating in your home. The thermostat in your hall or living room senses the temperature. If the temperature falls below a certain pre-set level, the thermostat activates the oil-fired or gas furnace to produce more heat. When the temperature rises to or above the pre-set level, the thermostat turns the furnace off or reduces its heat production.

Look upon the thyroid gland as the furnace and the pituitary gland—or certain cells in it —as the thermostat. The pituitary gland is the size of a grape and lies at the base of your brain. It secretes many different hormones but the one we are interested in now is the thyroid-stimulating hormone, also known as TSH or thyrotrophin. TSH passes into the bloodstream and activates the thyroid gland to release the stored thyroid hormones, to manufacture more of them, and to extract more iodine from the blood to do so. As a result of this stimulation of the thyroid cells the level of the thyroid hormones in the bloodstream rises. The cells in the pituitary that secrete TSH sense this, just as your thermostat senses the rise in the temperature in your sitting room. When the level of the thyroid hormones reaches a certain point, the secretion of TSH by the pituitary is reduced and the furnace (the thyroid gland) stops working so hard. This is what is called a feed-back control mechanism (Fig. 2).

The pituitary gland is very sensitive to the levels of the thyroid hormones circulating in the blood. It is also responsive to other signals from higher in the brain, particularly from another little gland called the hypothalamus.

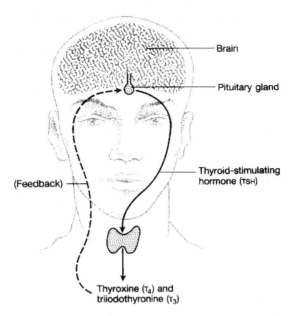

Brain

Pituitary gland

Thyroid-stimulating
hormone (TSH)

(Feedback)

Thyroxine (T₄) and
triiodothyronine (T₃)

Figure 2 Mechanism controlling the secretion by the thyroid gland of thyroxine (T_4) and triiodothyronine (T_3). As the levels of T_4 and T_3 rise in the bloodstream, the secretion of the thyroid-stimulating hormone (TSH) from the pituitary gland is reduced or switched off (feedback control mechanism). As the levels of T_4 and T_3 fall, the pituitary gland secretes more TSH so that activity of the thyroid gland is increased.

How do the thyroid hormones get around in the bloodstream?

The answer is that both hormones are mainly carried loosely attached to certain proteins in the blood. In a sense you can look upon the hormones as coal being carried in an open coal truck (the hormone-carrying proteins). More than 99.9 per cent of the two hormones are transported in this way, bound to the carrier proteins. However, while attached to these carrier proteins the hormones are biologically inactive, just as you cannot use the coal in a coal truck unless you first take it out of the truck. Only when the thyroid hormones are freed from their protein binding do they become biologically active at the cellular level. Some of the hormones, less than a fraction of one per cent of the total, are not attached to the carrier proteins and are floating free, as it were, in the water of your blood. These unattached hormones are biologically active.

You will hear more about this later because the protein-bound and the so-called free hormones are important when it comes to measuring the levels of T_4 and T_3 in the blood. Sometimes changes occur in the carrier proteins so that more, or less, of the hormone is protein-bound with less, or more, of the hormone being free, unbound, and biologically active.

Questions and Answers

Q.1   What is the thyroid gland?
A.   It is a small gland that controls the activity of your body cells.

Q.2   Where is the thyroid gland?
A.   It lies in the front of your neck in the position where a man knots his tie.

Q.3   What does the thyroid do?
A.   It produces the thyroid hormones which are chemical messengers sent to the rest of the body.

Q.4   What controls the output of thyroid hormones?
A.   The output depends upon the level of thyroid hormones in your blood. If the level falls, the pituitary gland puts out more thyroid-stimulating hormone (TSH) which stimulates the gland to make more hormones and release them into the bloodstream.

2
Things that go wrong with the thyroid gland

Certain conditions afflict only the thyroid gland and do not, indeed cannot, occur elsewhere in any other tissue or organ in your body. For example, overactivity of the thyroid (hyperthyroidism), in which too much hormone is secreted, and underactivity (hypothyroidism), in which too little hormone is secreted, are disorders peculiar and specific to the thyroid and produce characteristic symptoms. Certain other disorders of the thyroid gland, on the other hand, such as infections, inflammation, and cancer, are not so unique to the thyroid because similar changes may occur in other organs. Nevertheless, the symptoms and the clinical picture induced by infection, inflammation, or cancer are strongly coloured by the fact that the disease process is taking place in the thyroid.

Let us take a brief preliminary look at some of the common disorders that may affect the thyroid gland.

Increase in size

Enlargement of the thyroid gland from any cause is called a goitre. The whole gland may be enlarged uniformly, or only one part of it. A goitre may vary in size from a thyroid gland that feels slightly larger than normal, to one that is clearly visible (Fig. 3a) and on to one that is a large lump the size of an orange (Fig. 3b).

Many disorders of the thyroid gland may make it bigger. The enlargement may be associated with a normal output

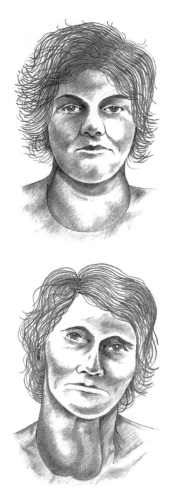

Figure 3 (a) A medium-sized goitre. (b) A large nodular goitre in a patient living in an iodine-deficient area of the world.

of thyroid hormones, and the patient is then said to be euthyroid. The goitre may be associated with an increased secretion of thyroid hormone, and the patient is then said to be hyperthyroid. Or it may be associated with a decreased deficient output and the patient is then hypothyroid. From this you will see that the size of the thyroid gland bears little relationship to its secretory activity or function. A small goitre or even a thyroid gland of normal size may produce excess thyroid hormones, whereas a large goitre may be associated with deficient secretion.

Goitres are usually painless but in some conditions the gland hurts and is tender on pressure. If sufficiently large the goitre may cause some discomfort on swallowing. If a goitre becomes very large it is not only cosmetically unsightly but it may press on the windpipe and cause difficulty with breathing. It may also press on the veins in the neck carrying blood to the heart from the face and brain and cause a sense of fullness in the head.

Slight enlargement of the thyroid gland is so common in women at the time of puberty and during pregnancy that it is looked upon as normal. Do not be self-conscious if you have a small goitre, which seldom is as unsightly as you may think. In fact not so long ago a small goitre was considered a mark of beauty, as shown by many of the portraits of elegant women painted by the prolific Dutch court painter Lely (1619–80).

The cause of a goitre must be sought and the necessary steps taken to prevent it from becoming larger. A more detailed account of goitres in given is Chapters 10 and 11.

Autoimmune disorders

The thyroid gland is particularly prone to autoimmune disorders, but first we must explain what an autoimmune disorder is.

What is an autoimmune disorder?

All of us have an immune system which protects us from infection with commonly encountered bacteria and viruses. A baby inherits some of its immunity from its mother, particularly if the baby is breast-fed. Later in life the baby meets these infections and develops what is usually a life-long immunity to them. How does this immune system work?

In the blood are certain white corpuscle cells called lymphocytes which are on the look-out for the 'foreign' proteins that occur in micro-organisms and viruses— 'foreign' because the proteins are not a constituent of the normal individual. The lymphocytes spot that the proteins are 'foreign' and develop chemical substances, called antibodies, to neutralize them. The situation is like that of soldiers becoming aware that foreign enemy troops have penetrated their defences. Just as the soldiers will round up the enemy troops to disarm or kill them, so the lymphocytes react by producing antibodies that neutralize or kill the invading micro-organisms comprised of 'foreign' proteins.

Foreign proteins of any sort are looked upon as invading enemies, and antibodies are formed against them. This is why there are problems when a tissue, such as skin, or an organ, such as a kidney or the heart, essentially made of protein, is transplanted from one person to another. The lymphocytes of the recipient of the transplant look upon the donated tissue or organ as 'foreign', which it is. The recipient's white cells form antibodies which attack the transplant and, without special intervention by the doctor, would destroy it. This rejection by the recipient is one of the major problems in transplant surgery.

In autoimmune disorders, for reasons we do not yet fully understand, the lymphocytes get the idea that some tissue or organ in your body does not belong to you; it should not be there; it is 'foreign'. Antibodies are produced that mount an attack on the 'self' in the mistaken belief that the tissue is 'foreign'. Because these antibodies attack the 'self' they are called autoantibodies. It is like a group of soldiers mistakenly thinking that the troops serving alongside them in the same regiment belong to the enemy.

In the case of autoimmune thyroid disorders, the lymphocytes produce antibodies that react with the cells, or certain constituents of the cells, of the thyroid gland. The presence and strength of these antibodies can be measured in your blood.

Some antibodies are destructive and kill off the thyroid cells. Other antibodies stimulate the thyroid cells to produce too much thyroid hormone. Occasionally destructive and stimulating antibodies occur together or operate one after the other so that after having an overactive thyroid gland for a time the patient becomes thyroid deficient.

Hyperthyroidism

An increase above the normal level of thyroxine or of triiodothyronine, but usually both, causes thyroid overactivity (hyperthyroidism or thyrotoxicosis). The most common cause of this is an autoimmune disease called Graves' disease, named after the Dublin physician, Dr Robert Graves, who described the condition in three young women in 1835. In the English-speaking world autoimmune hyperthyroidism still bears his name. In Europe, however, Graves' disease is known as Basedow's disease after Carl von Basedow, who published a very clear account of the condition in 1840, which often is characterized by a small goitre, palpitations of the heart, and changes in the eyes.

In hyperthyroidism, or thyrotoxicosis as it is also called, the metabolism of the cells in the body is increased. The clinical picture varies somewhat depending upon your age but the most common features are a rapid heart rate and palpitations, an increase in bowel activity causing frequent loose motions or diarrhoea, and an increased metabolism, causing loss of weight. Graves' disease, in which antibodies stimulate the thyroid cells to secrete excess thyroid hormones, is considered in more detail in Chapter 4. The commonly associated eye changes are discussed in Chapter 5. Other less common causes of hyperthyroidism are dealt with in Chapter 6.

Hypothyroidism

Underactivity of the thyroid gland may have many different causes and is discussed in Chapters 7 and 8. Worldwide, iodine deficiency is much the most common cause of thyroid deficiency at any age, but in the Western world the most common cause of hypothyroidism is chronic autoimmune thyroiditis, also known as lymphadenoid or chronic lymphocytic goitre, or Hashimoto's disease after the Japanese surgeon who described the appearance of the gland in 1912 (Chapter 7).

In hypothyroidism the body cells work sluggishly. The heart rate slows, the bowels are sluggish leading to constipation, the skin becomes dry and thickened, the voice is deeper and croaky, and you become intolerant of cold. The clinical features are discussed in detail in Chapter 8.

Thyroiditis

Infection or inflammation of the thyroid gland is not uncommon. The usual cause of obvious acute thyroid inflammation is a virus. This subacute viral thyroiditis, also called de Quervain's thyroiditis after a Swiss physician who first described it, is 'subacute' because the degree of discomfort in the neck due to inflammation of the thyroid gland is usually not very severe but it tends to persist for several weeks or months if left untreated. The gland hurts and is tender to the touch; swallowing may be painful. Subacute viral thyroiditis is discussed in Chapter 9. The inflammation may temporarily cause excessive amounts of thyroid hormones to leach out of the gland and for some weeks you will suffer from thyroid overactivity (thyrotoxicosis).

Sometimes a virus infection or an autoimmune reaction causes no discomfort at all in the thyroid gland, and the associated hyperthyroidism is then attributed to 'silent thyroiditis' which is discussed in Chapters 13 and 14.

Very rarely the thyroid is attacked by a bacterial microorganisms, such as the common streptococcus that may cause an acute sore throat, by a staphylococcus that commonly causes boils (furunculosis), or by the tubercle bacillus.

Cancer

Among disorders of the thyroid gland, cancer is rare; and among malignant growths in the body as a whole, it is even rarer. Most thyroid cancers are well differentiated; this means that the cells that make up the cancer continue to look like relatively normal thyroid cells under the microscope. These malignant cells do not usually multiply rapidly and hence the tumour does not grow rapidly. Not only do the cancer cells look rather like normal thyroid cells, but they often behave like them. For instance, they usually remain responsive to the action of thyroid-stimulating hormone and they continue to extract iodine from the bloodstream. This means that in addition to surgical removal of the growth, which is the usual initial treatment, any remaining malignant cells can be eliminated by treatment with radioactive iodine (Chapter 12). Provided the condition is diagnosed early, the treatment of a differentiated thyroid cancer is usually very successful.

Questions and Answers

Q.1   If I develop a goitre, does it mean I've got cancer?

A.   Certainly not. Thyroid cancer is very rare and there are a great many more common benign conditions that cause enlargement of the thyroid.

Q.2   What is an autoimmune disease?

A.   It is a disorder of your immune system which gets the mistaken idea that some organ or tissue in your body does not belong to you: it is 'foreign' and should be got rid of.

Q.3 In an autoimmune disease, how does my body try to get rid of the allegedly 'foreign' cells?

A. Certain chemicals, autoantibodies, are developed that attack the supposedly 'foreign' cells (see also p. 37).

Q.4 Are the autoantibodies always destructive?

A. No, sometimes they can stimulate your thyroid gland to increased secretory activity, as happens in Graves' disease.

3
How the doctor finds out what is wrong

To find out what is wrong with your thyroid gland, your doctor will first wish to hear all about your symptoms. Do tell your doctor everything. Do not omit any symptom just because *you* think it is irrelevant; it may not be. After listening to you, the doctor will probably need to ask you a number of questions, either for you to expand on certain things you have found wrong with yourself or to discuss matters that you may not have mentioned.

Then you will be examined. In addition to the general physical examination, particular attention will be given to your weight (and height in the case of children), your pulse rate, and the findings in your neck.

If you have any eye symptoms, the distance between the front of each eye and edge of the bony socket in which the eye lies may be painlessly measured in clinics that specialize in thyroid disorders (Fig. 14, p. 66). Additional eye tests may be arranged and photographs taken of your neck and of your eyes.

Almost certainly, blood and other tests will be carried out. These can be divided into two main groups:

1. Tests to tell whether your thyroid is putting out the correct amount, or too little or too much, of the thyroid hormones.

2. Tests designed to give information as to what is wrong with your thyroid gland. These will help to answer such questions as:
   • Why is my thyroid gland enlarged?

- Why is my gland overactive (or underactive)?
- Why have I got a lump in my thyroid; is it serious?
- Why is the front of my neck so sore?

Direct tests of thyroid function

Over the years many different methods have been used to determine whether your thyroid gland is making the right amount of thyroid hormones. Modern tests are carried out on a small sample of blood taken from a vein, and usually the results are available within a few days. Regrettably it must, however, be admitted that no one single test of thyroid function is always 100 per cent diagnostically reliable, because a result that is too high or too low may occur for a number of different reasons (see Glossary, p. 167).

Thyroid-stimulating hormone (TSH) level

With modern techniques, normal, high, and low levels of TSH can be measured very accurately. Of course, the level of TSH is not exactly the same in every healthy person, and the normal or reference range is that which is found in 95 per cent of healthy people. This range will vary from one laboratory to another depending upon the precise technical procedure used and the normal population being studied by that laboratory.

The Underactive gland. In hypothyroidism when the secretion of thyroid hormones is reduced, the pituitary gland responds by secreting more TSH in order to increase the activity of the flagging thyroid. The TSH level is increased roughly in proportion to the decrease in the thyroxine blood level. Thus in established hypothyroidism, with all the characteristic clinical symptoms and signs, the TSH level is very high. When the degree of thyroid under-activity is more marginal, before any florid evidence of it may have appeared and the thyroxine level is at or just below its lower normal range, the TSH will be increased to a lesser degree, but this is of great help in confirming that the thyroid gland is having to struggle. Indeed experience has shown that in the diagnosis of a failing thyroid, the TSH level is the most sensitive test for detecting this.

The Overactive gland. When the thyroid is overactive and increased amounts of thyroid hormones are being secreted, the pituitary gland is switched off by the feedback mechanism (p. 6 and Fig. 2). The TSH level falls below normal. This test is therefore of value in helping to confirm a diagnosis of hyperthyroidism, when the TSH will be below the bottom of the reference range and may even be undetectable. However, low levels of TSH may also occur in circumstances other than hyperthyroidism (see Glossary, p. 179).

Thyroxine (T_4) level

Both the total amount of thyroxine in the bloodstream, which is largely bound to carrier proteins, and the free thyroxine, which is the tiny amount floating free in the water of your blood, can be measured. Some laboratories measure the total T_4 and others the free T_4. The advantages and disadvantages of the two methods are discussed in the Glossary (p. 171 and 180).

Hyperthyroidism. Raised levels of thyroxine occur in most cases of hyperthyroidism but sometimes only the level of triiodothyronine (T_3) is raised. The more severe the overactivity of the gland, the higher are these blood hormone levels.

Hypothyroidism. Reduced levels of thyroxine occur in most cases of hypothyroidism, but not always to a marked degree in the early stages (see Chapter 8).

The main trouble with measuring the total thyroxine compared with the free thyroxine level is that the former is influenced so much by the level of the carrier proteins to which the T_4 is loosely attached, and may not truly reflect your thyroid status. Most thyroidologists prefer to measure the free thyroxine. Sometimes an additional test is used in conjunction with the total thyroxine to make allowance for variations in the proteins that transport thyroxine in the bloodstream. This test is used in conjunction with the total T_4 to derive the so-called free thyroxine index (FTI). This is an indirect indication of the free thyroxine level but is now becoming obsolete.

Free thyroxine index

The free thyroxine index reflects that amount of thyroxine which is unattached to protein and is free in the blood, in much the same way as the free T_4 test does. It is the unbound thyroxine that we really want to know about because the free thyroxine determines your thyroid status. It is for this reason that in most centres measurement of the free T_4 is now used in preference to the total serum thyroxine and the free thyroxine index tests.

Triiodothyronine (T_3) level

Both the total (protein-bound) and the free T_3 levels can be measured. High levels of both occur if you have an overactive thyroid. In some patients with hyperthyroidism the T_3 level rises some weeks or months earlier than does the thyroxine level. Indeed, there are some patients with thyrotoxicosis with a raised T_3 level who never develop a raised thyroxine level. Thus if you have symptoms and signs indicative of hyperthyroidism and a low TSH level but a normal level of thyroxine, the finding of a high T_3 (total or free) will explain the situation, which is known as T_3-toxicosis.

In the diagnosis of hypothyroidism the T_3 level is much less useful because the failing thyroid gland finds it easier to produce triiodothyronine than thyroxine. Thus the level of T_3 falls later and more slowly than does the thyroxine and may be normal in patients with quite severe hypothyroidism.

Low levels of T_3 may also occur in patients suffering from many physical and psychiatric illnesses quite unrelated to the thyroid gland. This is called the 'sick euthyroid' syndrome, in which much of the thyroxine is converted to the inactive form of T_3 known as reversed T_3, because it is the mirror image of the active form and its formation is increased in the sick euthyroid syndrome. The T_3 level gradually returns to normal as the patient recovers (p. 154).

Combined tests

A great deal can be said for assessing the secretory activity of the thyroid from two different angles by doing two different *types* of thyroid function tests:

- the level of the thyroid hormones on the one hand; and
- the secretion of TSH on the other.

Even when the diagnosis is obvious, your doctor is likely to assess the situation by measuring *either* the total or preferably the free T_4 (and sometimes in suspected hyperthyroidism also the total or free T_3) *and* the TSH level if you are suspected of having overactivity or underactivity of the thyroid gland.

Table 1 summarizes some of the results that may be obtained by measuring the free thyroxine, the free triiodothyronine, and the TSH levels.

Indirect tests of thyroid function

A number of indirect tests may be used to assess thyroid secretory function.

Radio-iodine uptake

This test is based upon the uptake by the thyroid gland of one of the radioactive isotopes of iodine. In hyperthyroidism the production of excess amounts of the thyroid hormones requires more of the essential raw material, namely iodine. Hence the thyroid has to take more iodine out of the bloodstream for hormone synthesis. Conversely, in hypothyroidism less iodine, or radioactive iodine, is

Table 1 A summary of some common results of tests of thyroid secretory function and their significance

Free T$_4$ level	Free T$_3$ level	TSH level	Significance
High	High	Low	Hyperthyroidism or excess treatment with T$_4$
Normal	High	Low	Early hyperthyroidism; T$_3$-toxicosis
Normal	Normal	Normal	Normal euthyroid
Normal or slightly high	Normal	Normal or slightly low	Euthyroid on treatment with T$_4$
Normal or low	Normal	Normal or low	Generalized ill-health; 'sick euthyroid' syndrome
Low or normal	Normal	High	Subclinical or mild hypothyroidism
Low	Normal or low	High	Hypothyroidism

trapped because less than normal amounts of thyroid hormones are being made.

The uptake of radio-iodine is measured by you being given an injection of radioactive isotope or by you taking it orally. The radioactivity in your thyroid is measured with a counter placed over your neck after 2–6 hours if you are suspected of having an overactive gland, and after 24–48 hours if you are suspected of having an underactive one.

This is an indirect method of assessing the production of thyroid hormones. The situation is similar to that in a motorcar factory in which iodine is akin to the steel going into the plant. It can be argued that the more raw material (in this case steel) that goes into the factory the more cars come out the other end. Over a prolonged period of time this would probably be true, but in the short term all sorts of fallacies may arise. The factory might be stockpiling steel and holding it in store without increasing car production. The factory might be making the usual number of cars but storing them in the plant and not releasing them for distribution. Similarly with iodine, an increase in uptake may indicate stockpiling, perhaps because the thyroid gland has been starved of iodine for a time. Thus increased uptake cannot invariably be equated with increased production of thyroid hormones. Even though the thyroid may be capable of normal hormone synthesis, the uptake of iodine will be suppressed if you are taking T_4 or T_3 by mouth because such medication will depress the secretion of TSH by the pituitary and the thyroid will be in an inactive, resting state.

One of the most instructive examples of a possibly misleading result being obtained by measuring the uptake of radio-iodine is in sub-acute viral thyroiditis (Chapter 9). In this condition the thyroid cells are disorganized by the inflammation caused by a virus. They cannot work properly and hence the uptake of iodine is zero. However, the inflammatory process causes preformed thyroid hormones stored in the gland to be released into the circulation so that the symptoms and signs of hyperthyroidism develop.

Various slightly different isotopes of iodine are used, often a tracer amount of ^{131}I but sometimes ^{123}I or ^{132}I because they have a shorter radioactive life than ^{131}I and they decay more quickly, hence causing less irradiation to your body in general. They are preferred for studies in children and whenever repeated tests are made. If you are given these isotopes in trace amounts, you can confidently be reassured that the irradiation hazard is negligible but even so they will not be used if you are pregnant because the radio-isotope will enter the thyroid gland of your baby.

For reasons of convenience another isotope called technetium (^{99m}Tc) is often used in place of iodine isotopes. This is taken up by the thyroid cells in the same way as iodine is trapped but it is not incorporated in the making of the thyroid hormones. Technetium and the iodine isotopes now find their main use in determining what is wrong with the thyroid gland (p. 27) rather than for assessing its secretory function.

Ankle reflex relaxation time

The speed of the tendon reflexes, such as the well-known reaction when the tendon just below your knee-cap is tapped with a hammer, is influenced by the level of thyroid hormones. In practice, the ankle reflex, and in particular the time it takes to relax after contraction, as judged by tapping on the Achilles tendon at the back of your heel, is the one used, and the speed of the movement of your foot may be recorded with an electronic device. The time for the muscle to relax is often much slower in hypothyroidism and it is quicker than normal in hyperthyroidism. This test is influenced, however, by factors other than the circulating levels of the thyroid hormones. Although it can be useful in assessing your response to treatment, it is of limited value in the primary assessment of thyroid function.

Cholesterol

The level of cholesterol, a particular type of fat in the blood, is influenced by the amount of thyroid hormones secreted. In hypothyroidism the cholesterol is usually substantially raised above normal and in hyperthyroidism it is often low. However, cholesterol level is influenced by many other factors and variations from normal in thyroid disease may occur only when the degree of disordered secretory function is quite marked and of long standing.

Tests to determine the cause of thyroid disease

Having decided that your thyroid is not functioning normally, your doctor will need to find out exactly why it has gone wrong. For instance you may have a goitre but thyroid secretory function is normal. Why then have you developed a goitre? Equally, if your gland is underactive or overactive, your doctor must find out exactly why.

It is not enough to decide that you are, for example, hypothyroid by finding that the free thyroxine level is low and the TSH level is high. The next question to be asked and answered is 'what has gone wrong with this thyroid gland to make it underactive?' This may be obvious if you have been previously treated for hyperthyroidism with radio-iodine or by surgery. In less obvious cases there are many possible explanations, such as iodine deficiency or more probably Hashimoto's disease.

Investigations will help to decide if a lump in your thyroid gland is a hollow cyst or a solid nodule, and whether it is benign (non-cancerous) or malignant (Chapters 11 and 12).

It is also necessary to determine whether hyperthyroidism is due to an autoimmune process that induces the whole gland to secrete excess thyroid hormones (Graves' disease) or to temporary thyroiditis, or whether it is due to a localized area of overactive cells producing too much hormone (a toxic adenoma). These distinctions are important because they have a significant bearing on the right treatment for you.

Hence the investigations discussed in this section are directed at finding out why the thyroid is behaving abnormally. Not all these tests are likely to be required or necessary and the order in which they are done will vary according to what your doctor suspects has gone wrong.

Thyroid antibodies

As explained on page 12 in Chapter 2, antibodies may develop in your body which act on the cells of the thyroid gland in different ways. Detection of these antibodies and assessment of their level may be crucial in deciding what is wrong with you.

Thyroid-inhibiting antibodies. A variety of different antibodies may impair thyroid function. The two most common are the thyroglobulin and the microsomal antibodies. The most important is the microsomal, also known as the thyroid peroxidase (TPO) antibody. This antibody is cytotoxic, which means that it destroys thyroid cells. It is usually found in the blood of patients with Hashimoto's disease and is directly responsible for the gradual destruction of the thyroid with the subsequent development of hypothyroidism. This autoimmune destruction is a slow process and takes place over many months and years. At the present time we do not have a safe and effective way of arresting the destructive process, but the knowledge that this antibody is present will ensure that a careful eye is kept on you so that replacement therapy with thyroxine is given as soon as, or even before, the thyroid ceases to secrete an adequate amount of hormones.

It is also important to know that you have an autoimmune disorder of the thyroid gland because this is sometimes associated sooner or later with other autoimmune diseases (Chapter 15). Thus your doctor may wish, for example, to check for the presence of an antibody that destroys certain cells in the stomach, the secretion of which is responsible for the absorption of vitamin B_{12}— a vitamin essential for the making of the red corpuscles in your blood. If this antibody is found to be present, a check must be kept on your haemoglobin level and injections of vitamin B_{12} given at the earliest evidence of anaemia developing (p. 159).

Thyroid-stimulating-antibodies. Antibodies that increase thyroid activity are the probable cause of Graves' disease. These thyroid-stimulating substances can be detected in about 90 per cent of patients with Graves' disease and occur also in 60 per cent of patients who have the eye complications of Graves' disease but are not yet thyrotoxic (Chapter 5). The same antibodies may also occur in those patients with hypothyroidism caused by Hashimoto's disease who have a transient episode of hyperthyroidism ('Hashitoxicosis', p. 84), or alternating episodes of hyper- and hypothyroidism.

Radio-isotope thyroid scan

In this investigation you are given a radio-isotope, either technetium or iodine, that is taken up by your thyroid gland. The gland becomes temporarily radioactive and this is charted by a counter placed over your neck. The amount of radioactive material to which you are exposed is very small and you need have no fears as to the amount of irradiation your body receives. A record of the uptake in your neck (the scintigram) may be charted on X-ray film or on paper in colour, as shown in Fig. 4 (reproduced here in black and white).

A normal thyroid isotope scan will show that the gland is located in the right place. It will show the right and left lobes to be of approximately equal size. It may not always show the isthmus. The uptake of the isotope is uniform throughout both lobes but the radioactivity is greater in the centre of each lobe than at the edges because there is more thyroid tissue in the middle of the lobe.

If the thyroid gland does not develop properly or its descent into the neck from its origins at the base of the tongue is abnormal (see Chapter 1), the scintigram will show little radioactivity in the usual place but the activity

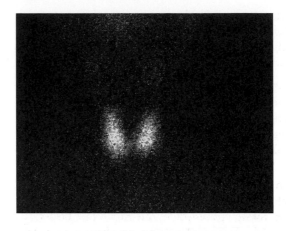

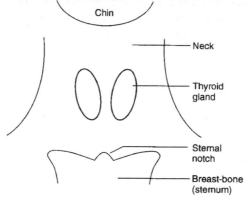

Figure 4 Technetium isotope scan of a normal thyroid gland. The outline of the gland is clearly shown. The patient's right lobe is slightly larger than the left. The degree of uptake of the isotope is greatest in the centre of each lobe, where there is most thyroid tissue. The 'sternal notch' is the small hollow at the upper end of the breast-bone.

may be located high in the neck, under the chin. These findings are mainly of importance when seeking the cause of hypothyroidism in a baby or child.

When the thyroid descends too far, the scan will usually

show some activity in the lower part of the neck but most is found behind the upper part of the breast-bone (a retro-sternal thyroid) or, more rarely, lower down in the chest (a mediastinal thyroid).

Hyperthyroidism. When there is overactivity of the thyroid the scan may show one of four different appearances, depending upon the cause:

- In Graves' disease the whole gland is overactive, and the scan shows high activity uniformly throughout both lobes. Usually the lobes are enlarged, but not always.

- When the thyrotoxicosis is caused by overactivity in just one clump of cells (a toxic adenoma), the radioactivity is almost totally confined to this area of hyperactivity (Fig. 5). This is referred to as a 'hot' nodule because of the excess uptake of isotope in this one area. The rest of the gland takes up little or no isotope and is 'cold' because it is inactive as a result of the excess thyroid hormones formed by the hot nodule depressing the pituitary secretion of TSH through the normal feedback mechanism.

- In a multinodular toxic goitre the isotope uptake is largely confined to a number of different areas which vary in size and in their 'hotness'. Thus the scan shows multiple 'hot' nodules separated by areas of relatively inactive 'cold' tissue.

- When hyperthyroidism is caused by viral thyroiditis, the working of the thyroid gland is so disrupted that it temporarily ceases to function and the scan shows very little or no uptake. The thyrotoxicosis is due to preformed thyroid hormones being discharged from the inflamed gland. With recovery from the inflammation, the gland will show a normal uptake again some months after the initial illness.

Because the treatment of these different causes of hyperthyroidism is not the same, it is important that the distinction is made. Of course an isotope scan is not

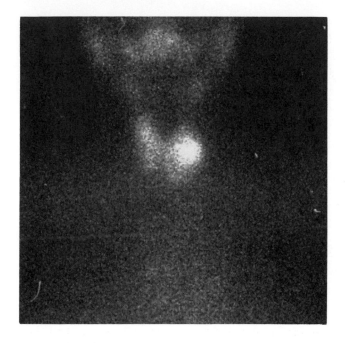

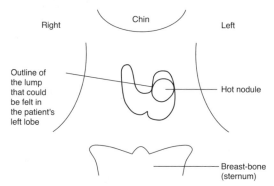

Figure 5 Technetium isotope scan of a thyroid gland
containing a toxic adenoma. The 'hot' nodule in the patient's
left lobe takes up most of the isotope, and there is little radioactivity in the other lobe because it is inactive as a result of T_4
from the nodule suppressing the secretion of TSH from the
pituitary gland (see text).

necessary in every hyperthyroid patient because the diagnosis may be obvious if you have thyrotoxicosis together
with the eye signs of Graves' ophthalmopathy. In some
cases of viral thyroiditis the diagnosis is also obvious to your
doctor from your history of a 'flu-like illness followed by
pain and tenderness in the thyroid and the symptoms and
signs of thyrotoxicosis. However, some cases of thyroiditis
are not associated with an obvious 'flu-like illness and the
thyroid gland is not painful (so-called 'silent thyroiditis',
p. 151).

Nodular or lumpy goitres.   Isotope scans can be helpful in
deciding the nature of a lump or lumps in one or both lobes
of your thyroid gland. Quite often we see a patient who has
noticed a lump in her neck, perhaps the size of a grape,
which may be completely painless. On examination the
lump is found to be part of the thyroid gland: on swallowing
it moves with the rest of the gland which feels perfectly normal. A scan with ^{131}I, ^{123}I, or ^{99m}Tc may show that the nodule does not take up the isotope and is 'cold' (Fig. 6). This
makes it slightly more likely that the nodule could be malignant but in fact most, about 80 per cent, of 'cold' nodules
when biopsied prove not to be malignant (see below).
Sometimes an isotope scan done to investigate what
appears on examination to be a solitary nodule shows that
not only is the nodule 'cold' but that there are other 'cold'
areas in the rest of the gland which your doctor cannot feel.
This is helpful because it shows that you have multiple
'cold' nodules, not a solitary one, and this makes it even less
likely that malignant change has occurred.

Thus isotope scanning with radio-iodine may be useful
in the assessment of patients with thyroid lumps (Chapter
11) and is invaluable in the management of those with
thyroid cancer (Chapter 12).

Ultrasound scan

This technique, also sometimes called a sonogram or
echogram, is painless. Some jelly is spread over your neck

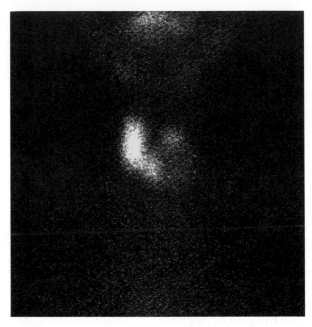

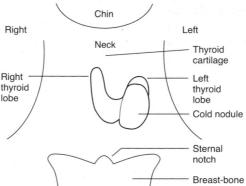

Figure 6 Technetium scan of a thyroid gland containing a 'cold' nodule. The nodule in the lower part of the left lobe could easily be seen and felt. There is no radioactivity in this module which is, therefore, 'cold'. Some radioactivity can be seen in the area of the chin because the isotope has also been taken up in the salivary glands. (Note that 'right' and 'left' in the diagram refer to the patient's right and left.)

and a probe moved backwards and forwards across your thyroid gland. This probe sends an inaudible painless 'sound' wave through the skin into your thyroid gland which is reflected back to a receiver in the probe.

As the probe is moved from side to side a pattern emerges which is recorded (Fig. 7) just as when this technique is used for locating a submarine or a wreck on the seabed. The ultrasound will show the size of your thyroid gland, whether a lump is a solid nodule or a hollow cyst filled with fluid and whether there is a single nodule or several.

Biopsy

A biopsy is the removal of a small piece of thyroid tissue for examination under the microscope. This is helpful because a careful study of the cells can often tell your doctor what exactly is wrong; for example whether a nodule is benign or malignant. A fine-needle aspiration is a virtually painless procedure carried out in a few minutes on an outpatient basis. Thyroid tissue or fluid containing some cells is sucked through a fine needle into a syringe.

You lie on a couch with your neck stretched back. There is a slight prick as a fine needle is inserted into the thyroid gland and a small sliver of tissue or fluid removed. Most doctors do not first inject a local anaesthetic because many patients find this unnecessary. After the fine-needle aspiration a small adhesive dressing is put over the puncture mark in your neck and you can safely go home after a short rest.

Unfortunately sometimes not enough tissue is obtained for the pathologist, who examines the cells, to make a firm diagnosis and sometimes the cells are not taken from the abnormal area. If there is continuing doubt, your doctor may advise you to have a repeat of the fine-needle aspiration or an operation, usually a hemithyroidectomy, which provides both a firm diagnosis and often a cure because the whole of the lump in question and the surrounding tissue are removed.

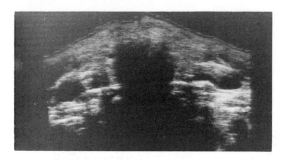

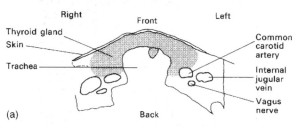

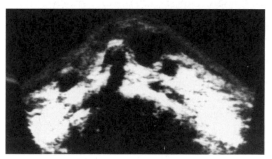

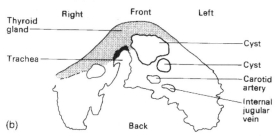

Figure 7 Ultrasound scans of the thyroid gland. (a) Normal. (b) A large and a small cyst in the left lobe are causing some thyroid enlargement.

X-rays

Conventional X-ray pictures may be taken to assess whether an enlarged thyroid gland is pressing on your windpipe or, if the goitre is larger on one side than the other, whether the windpipe is being displaced. A retrosternal or a mediastinal thyroid may first be discovered

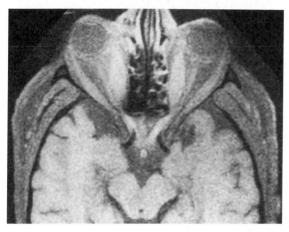

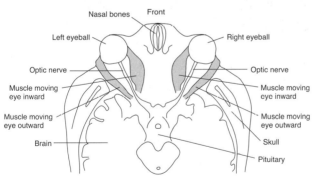

Figure 8 Magnetic resonance imaging (MRI) of a patient with impaired movements of the eyes and double vision. The eyeballs are clearly seen. The muscles that move the eyeballs inwards are much thicker than the normal muscles that move the eyes outward. (Note that the left and right orientations refer to the patient's left and right.)

only by chance from an X-ray of your chest taken for some other purpose. The nature of the retrosternal shadow may have to be confirmed by an isotope scan.

Computer-assisted tomography (a CAT or CT scan) or a magnetic resonance image (MRI) of the eyes and the bony sockets in which they lie is helpful to establish the nature of the eye changes that may be associated with Graves' disease, especially when these changes are confined to only one eye (Fig. 8).

Questions and Answers

Q.1   Will it hurt if I have a lot of blood tests done?

A.   It is unlikely that more than one or two samples of blood will be taken from a vein. Many different tests can be done on one sample. The taking of a blood sample is not usually painful.

Q.2   How will my doctor be able to tell if I have an overactive or an underactive thyroid?

A.   He may know from your symptoms and his findings on examination of you, but he will confirm the diagnosis by tests. It is likely that he will measure the levels of your thyroid-stimulating hormone (TSH) and your free T_4 to decide. He may also measure on the same sample your triiodothyronine (T_3) level if he thinks you are thyrotoxic.

Q.3   Is thyrotoxicosis the same thing as thyroid overactivity and hyperthyroidism?

A.   Yes. All these terms mean your thyroid is producing too much thyroid hormones.

Q.4   Does it mean I have cancer if I'm given a radioactive iodine test?

A.   Absolutely not.

Q.5   Are there several causes for overactivity or underactivity of the thyroid gland?

A.   Yes. In Chapters 5 and 6 the several causes of hyperthyroidism are discussed and in Chapter 8 the causes of hypothyroidism.

Q.6   What are thyroid auto-antibodies?

A.   They are chemicals produced in your body that influence your thyroid cells. They may destroy them (p. 12 and 26) or they may stimulate them (p. 13 and 27).

Q.7   If I have an isotope scan will it impair my fertility?

A.   No, it won't—not at all. The dose of irradiation is less than that given when a simple chest X-ray is done.

Q.8   Why is my hospital doctor so keen on finding out why I have an overactive thyroid gland?

A.   Because the most effective treatment differs with the cause.

Q.9   What does the doctor at the hospital mean when he says I'm to have a biopsy done as an outpatient?

A.   A fine-needle aspiration is a procedure to remove a small piece of tissue or fluid from your thyroid gland.

Q.10   Shouldn't I have had some X-rays taken?

A.   X-rays are of limited value in the investigation of thyroid disease, so don't worry if X-rays haven't been done.

4
Overactivity of the thyroid caused by Graves' disease

Overactivity of the thyroid gland, also known as hyperthyroidism or thyrotoxicosis, is a disease in which increased amounts of thyroid hormones are present in the bloodstream. Usually the levels of both thyroxine (T_4) and triiodothyronine (T_3) are increased above normal but in some people with thyroid overactivity only the T_3 level is raised, but the symptoms and the findings are just the same in this so-called T_3-toxicosis.

The causes of thyroid overactivity

The causes of overactivity of the thyroid are several (Table 2) but in practice more than 80 per cent of cases are due to the gland being subjected to excess stimulation by thyroid-stimulating antibodies. This condition is called Graves' disease or diffuse toxic goitre. It is 'diffuse' because the whole gland is overactive, as can be shown by an isotope scan (p. 28), and you are 'toxic' because you are ill—not sick because of some abnormal 'toxin' but because the cells of your body are being overstimulated by the increased levels of thyroid hormones circulating in your bloodstream.

In this chapter only Graves' disease is considered. The other less common causes of thyroid overactivity are discussed in Chapter 6.

Table 2   Some common causes of hyperthyroidism

- Graves' disease (diffuse toxic goitre)
- Multinodular toxic goitre
- Toxic adenoma
- Viral thyroiditis
- Hashitoxicosis
- Excessive dosage with T_4 or T_3

The cause of Graves' disease

Several factors are involved in the causation of Graves' disease:
- Often there is a familial or hereditary factor because autoimmune diseases of the thyroid gland and other organs or tissues tend to run in families (Chapter 15).
- The dietary intake of iodine is relevant because the disease often presents in the spring and summer after an increase of iodine intake during the previous months. In iodine-insufficient areas of the world, the incidence of Graves' disease may be temporarily increased if supplemental iodine is added to the diet.
- Females at all ages are some 10–15 times more likely than males to develop the condition. What triggers off the disease in those who are susceptible is unknown.
- In some instances Graves' disease seems to follow an emotional upset but it has not been possible to establish proof of such a cause-and-effect relationship.
- The fundamental cause of Graves' disease is the formation of antibodies that stimulate the thyroid cells to excess activity.

Who gets Graves' disease?

The disease is most common in women of all ages and may occur in younger children aged 5 or above and very rarely in a baby born of a mother who has, or has had in the past, Graves' disease.

What does it feel like?

The condition usually comes on insidiously, and it may be several months before you realize that you are ill, although rarely the outset is rapid over a few days or weeks. Tiredness is often an early symptom, to be followed by weight loss, palpitations or increased awareness of your heart beat, nervousness and particularly irritability so that you have 'a short fuse', and increased sweating. Looseness of the bowels is not uncommon and sometimes diarrhoea may be a prominent symptom, causing diagnostic problems unless the other features are detected.

You may feel hot and be uncomfortable in hot weather. You may complain that the central heating is set too high or throw off the bedclothes at night, yet your partner complains it is not *that* hot. Your skin may itch but there is no rash.

The tiredness gets worse and you may find yourself short of breath, particularly if you hurry while carrying shopping bags or climbing stairs. You may have a better than usual appetite; indeed you may be very hungry all the time. Even with this voracious appetite you may lose a lot of weight— up to 20 lb (9 kg)—but this is very variable. Your periods will tend to become less heavy and you may miss a period, or they may stop all together. If this happens, young women may wonder if they are pregnant but in fact they are likely to be infertile, a problem that corrects itself when the thyroid overactivity is brought under control.

You may not realize that you are physically weak. The upper muscles of your legs and arms are most likely to be affected. You may have difficulty in getting up from the squatting position without using your arms or find it hard to lift a heavy package down from a high shelf.

The older patient with Graves' disease. In patients aged 55 or over the typical features described above may be less

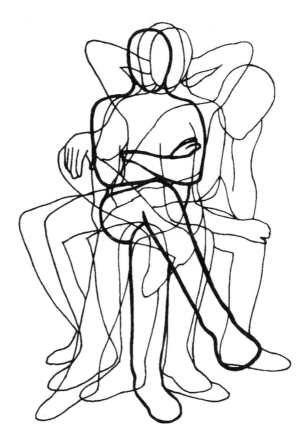

Figure 9 A representation of a patient with thyroid overactivity (thyrotoxicosis). Notice the restlessness. The patient cannot sit still and fidgets.

apparent and the brunt of the disease tends to fall upon the heart. The older patient often presents with shortness of breath, swollen ankles, and a fast, irregular heart beat which is called atrial fibrillation. Sleeping may be difficult unless you are propped up in bed and you may find by chance that it is easier to sleep sitting up in an armchair. The cause of this heart failure may not always be immediately apparent. Curiously some old people with Graves' disease become 'bloated' and lugubrious; they are slowed down and depressed (so-called 'apathetic hyperthyroidism', see p. 154).

Eye complications

The first thing you may notice is that something is wrong with your eyes. You may see in the mirror, or your friends may tell you, that one or both of your eyes has become starey. The upper lids are pulled upwards and the white of the eyes is more obvious (so-called 'lid retraction'). Because of this upper lid elevation your eyes appear larger (Fig. 10). The appearance is rather like an actress trying to convey fear or horror. This appearance may occur in thyroid overactivity from any cause, not only in Graves' disease. It improves as the overactivity of the thyroid gland is controlled or cured.

In Graves' disease, however, further eye troubles may arise, and these are discussed in Chapter 5.

Skin changes

You may notice that your skin is becoming thinner and more delicate, but this is seldom very obvious. Occasionally people with Graves' disease, and particularly those in whom the eye changes are marked, develop a curious change in the skin on their lower legs. Patches develop on the lower legs that are slightly reddened and thickened so that they stand up above the surrounding normal skin (Fig. 11). Hair growing in the affected areas becomes coarser. The areas tend to increase in size and new ones may appear on the top of your foot or on the big toe. This condition is called pretibial myxoedema. This term may be confusing because the word myxoedema is used to describe the generalized thickening of the skin seen in severe hypothyroidism (see Chapter 8).

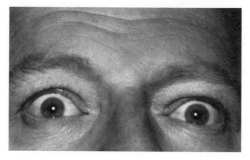

Figure 10 Lid retraction. Note how the upper eyelids are retracted so that the eyes have a staring quality and more of the white of the eyes than normal is visible.

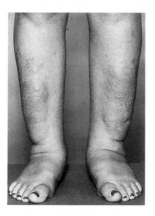 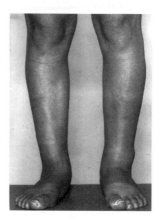

Figure 11 Pretibial myxoedema: (left) before treatment and (right) the appearance of the legs 18 months after the local application of corticosteroid ointment.

What does your doctor find when he examines you?

You are likely to be thin or at least show evidence of weight loss. You may be restless and anxious. You may not have noticed it, but it is hard for you to sit still and you probably fidget, plucking at your handbag or twiddling your fingers (Fig. 9, p. 42). Children tend to be clumsy and drop things; they may have grown faster than their contemporaries so that their height is greater than normal for their age.

Even on a cold day you will probably be lightly clad. Your hands are hot, the palms moist and your pulse bounding. Medical students are sometimes told, 'If your want to know the thyroid status of a young lady, you only have to hold her hand!' When your doctor asks you to hold out your arms in front of you and close your eyes, he or she may notice a fine tremor of your fingers. Your pulse rate is likely to be fast: this may be due in part to 'natural' nervousness on your part but in fact the fast rate is persistent and present even when you are asleep. Sometimes, particularly in the older patient, the heart beat is irregular due to atrial fibrillation.

Your thyroid gland may be normal in size but usually it is slightly enlarged, sometimes sufficiently so for a goitre to be your presenting complaint or noticed by your family or friends. Because it is overactive, the blood flow through the gland is increased and this may be audible as a swishing noise when your doctor puts a stethoscope on the front of your neck and asks you to stop breathing for a moment.

Often your eyes have a staring quality and this may be the first outward visible sign that alerts the doctor to what is wrong with you. Although you may be unaware that your muscles are weak, this may be obvious to your doctor. The most affected muscles are those round the shoulder and pelvic girdles. This weakness is more common in men than women. You may be surprised to find that you cannot raise your outstretched arms against the slight resistance of the doctor's hands or it may be difficult for you to get up from a squatting or lying position. While sitting on a chair you may not be able to hold one leg out horizontally for more than 25–30 seconds, whereas a normal person can do this for a minute or two.

Confirming the diagnosis

In its earliest stages, overactivity of the thyroid may not be easy to diagnose, or indeed be clinically evident. Later when the picture is more florid, it is easier. Your doctor has to distinguish thyroid overactivity from anxiety. Certainly in the younger person hyperthyroidism is virtually always accompanied by some feelings and evidence of anxiety, and the problem for the doctor is to distinguish anxiety alone from hyperthyroidism *plus* anxiety. The physical accompaniments of thyroid overactivity such as the weight loss, the fine tremor of the hands, and other evidence of increased metabolism are usually more pronounced than in uncomplicated anxiety, and laboratory tests will make the distinction.

The older hyperthyroid patient who predominantly presents with heart failure must be recognized as suffering from thyroid overactivity because with prompt treatment the outlook is good and often much better than for certain other forms of heart failure.

Laboratory tests usually give clear-cut confirmation of the diagnosis. The total or free T_4 and the total or free T_3 levels are raised above normal and the TSH level is depressed. In the early stages only your T_3 level may be raised but the TSH level will be depressed.

When the laboratory results are only marginally abnormal, little is lost if your doctor keeps you under observation and uses time as a diagnostic ally. The clinical picture and the laboratory tests will become clearer a month or two later.

Once a diagnosis of hyperthyroidism has been made by your doctor, he or she will wish to determine whether you have Graves' disease or one of the several other causes of thyrotoxicosis shown in Table 2 and discussed in Chapter 6.

The diagnosis of Graves' disease may be obvious if you have the characteristic eye changes associated with the condition and is even more likely if there is a history of thyroid disease in your family. It may be clear to your doctor from your history and the tenderness of your thyroid that you have not got Graves' disease but subacute viral thyroiditis (Chapter 9). Difficulties arise, however, if you have silent thyroiditis (p. 151). Examination of your neck may suggest that causes other than Graves' disease are the reason for the thyroid overactivity because instead of a uniform enlargement, one or more nodules are found in the gland.

In Graves' disease an isotope scan will show an increased uptake of the radio-isotope uniformly throughout both lobes. Furthermore, nearly all patients with Graves' disease have antimicrosomal (TPO) antibodies and thyroid-stimulating antibodies (TSAbs) in their blood, but this latter test is not universally available.

How will you be treated?

Curative treatment

If you have got Graves' disease, treatment is essential. In the old days about 20 per cent of untreated patients used to die and others ran a long fluctuating course with temporary remissions and relapses.

There are three main methods, not mutually exclusive, of treating Graves' disease. These are:

- antithyroid drugs, which suppress the ability of the thyroid gland to make thyroid hormones but induce a permanent cure in only about 50–60 per cent of patients;
- radio-iodine, ^{131}I, which is concentrated in the thyroid cells and, by irradiation, destroys them;
- surgical removal of most of the thyroid gland (subtotal thyroidectomy).

Which of these methods is used depends on several factors and circumstances which must be discussed between you and your doctor. The more important of these are:

- whether your hyperthyroidism is due to Graves' disease, or some other condition—all three methods can be used if you have got Graves' disease;

- your age;
- your sex;
- whether the thyroid gland is large or not, whether it is cosmetically unsightly, and whether it is causing compression or displacement of the windpipe;
- whether the thyroid gland is in the normal position or is lying behind the sternum;
- whether it is convenient for you to remain for 12–24 months under medical supervision for treatment with antithyroid drugs or whether you want a rapid, once-and-for-all cure;
- whether an experienced thyroid surgeon is available, because his results are likely to be better than those of a surgeon who does only occasional thyroid surgery;
- whether any eye complications are present and how severe they are;
- what previous treatment, if any, you have had. For example, if you have relapsed after a previous course of medical treatment, a second course of antithyroid drugs is less likely to achieve a permanent cure. If you have had surgery and thereafter relapsed, further surgery is contraindicated because the incidence of postoperative complications is too high;
- financial considerations. Surgical treatment with a week-long stay in hospital and the surgeon's and anaesthetist's fees is more expensive than treatment with radio-iodine. A year or 18 months of medical treatment is less expensive than surgery but more expensive than radio-iodine.

It is important for your peace of mind that you understand these considerations and appreciate the risks and the advantages and disadvantages of each form of treatment, which are further discussed later in this chapter.

Non-curative treatment

Two forms of treatment that will improve your symptoms and make you feel better, but will not permanently cure the overactivity of the thyroid gland, are important.

Beta-adrenergic blocking drugs, colloquially known as beta-blockers, reduce your sweating, the anxiety and restlessness, your palpitations and your fast heart-rate, and the tremor of your hands. Propranolol is commonly used for this purpose and in general is a very safe drug. However, it should not be taken by people who are prone to asthma. Propranolol has to be taken two or three times daily. There are other beta-blockers with slightly different modes of action and some of these, which can be given to asthma patients, are taken only once daily. Your doctor may decide that one of these is more appropriate for you than propranolol. The beta-blockers make you feel more comfortable until a proper cure has been achieved, but do not by themselves cure the condition. It is important for you to know that treatment with a beta-blocker should never be stopped suddenly, and you must not let yourself run out of tablets. When there is no more need for a beta-blocker, the dosage will be gradually reduced over a week or 10 days before the drug is finally stopped.

Iodine has a temporary suppressive effect on the thyroid gland by blocking the release of thyroid hormones, but this effect lasts for only 3 or 4 weeks. In the present-day management of hyperthyroidism iodine is mainly reserved for preparing you for surgery. You may be asked to take it in the form of drops of iodine (Lugol's iodine) in a little milk three times daily or as tablets of potassium iodide for 7–14 days before your operation. However, if you have been rendered euthyroid by medical treatment (see below) in preparation for elective surgery, iodine may not be needed.

Antithyroid drugs

A number of drugs suppress the synthesis of the thyroid hormones, reduce hormone production and will render you euthyroid. If the drug is given in too large a dose over too long a period of time you will become hypothyroid. Thus the dosage must be adjusted by your doctor, who may start with a large dose and later reduce it. Thereafter the dose is regulated by your clinical response and the blood level of your free thyroxine. However, once the hyperthyroidism has been brought under control, it is simpler for you to take a moderate dose of the antithyroid drug continuously and prevent hypothyroidism developing by taking in addition a small dose of thyroxine. This is called the block-and-replace regime, which works well in practice because it prevents you from having the ups and downs of being over- and underactive as may happen if the dosage of the antithyroid drug is constantly having to be adjusted. Another reason for giving a moderate dose of the antithyroid drug over a period of time, and using thyroxine to prevent thyroid underactivity developing, is that there is evidence that antithyroid drugs have a suppressive beneficial effect on the autoimmune process that is going on in your thyroid gland.

Although antithyroid drugs will certainly render you euthyroid, they may not provide a permanent cure. When the drug is stopped, the thyroid overactivity may gradually return over the next 3–24 months. In Graves' disease treatment for 12–18 months is associated with a permanent remission is about 50–60 per cent of patients. We are not sure why some people respond so favourably whereas others, in a matter months or years after stopping treatment, have a relapse of their thyroid overactivity, but this appears to be due to the persistence of thyroid-stimulating antibodies.

People who achieve a permanent remission often have only mild thyrotoxicosis, with a normal sized or only slightly enlarged gland and are treated from an early stage. Conversely those who have a large and vascular gland, are severely thyrotoxic, and whose treatment is started late are more liable to relapse when the antithyroid drug is stopped. But the size and vascularity of the gland and the severity of the hyperthyroidism are certainly not the only factors that determine the long-term response to antithyroid drugs. Your genetic constitution may be important and so also is the level of the thyroid-stimulating antibodies when the course of treatment has been completed. You must not look upon a relapse after medical treatment as a disaster. It simply prolongs the period of medical supervision until you are rendered euthyroid by subtotal thyroidectomy or by radio-iodine treatment. Which of these is used largely depends on your preferences. In many instances radio-iodine may prove the treatment of choice, depending on a variety of factors that will be discussed later.

People often ask why they cannot have another course of antithyroid drugs. They can, but experience has shown that failure to induce a permanent remission after the first course is likely to be followed by a relapse after a second or even a third course. Nor is protracted treatment with antithyroid drugs usually convenient because the intensity of the underlying disease fluctuates from time to time and this means you must be under continuous medical supervision.

Antithyroid drugs are best not used for treating people whose job precludes them from regular medical supervision, nor for those who cannot be relied upon to take their tablets regularly. If you want a quicker once-and-for-all cure choose radio-iodine or surgery. Surgery is indicated when the goitre is large and unsightly because the gland may not shrink in size very much after radio-iodine. Surgery is probably best when the goitre is retrosternal or when it is causing displacement or compression of the windpipe, particularly if of sufficient degree to interfere with your breathing (p. 57).

There is some evidence that radio-iodine treatment may release antibodies from the thyroid gland and these may aggravate severe eye complications. For this reason initial treatment with antithyroid drugs is often used to assess the effect on your eyes before deciding whether to go ahead with definitive curative treatment in the form of radio-iodine.

Age. Antithyroid drugs are used for those rare cases of hyperthyroidism that occur in new-born babies (Chapter 13). It is also the best treatment for children with Graves' disease, although they seldom experience a permanent remission. If you have a daughter with an overactive thyroid, antithyroid drugs with additional thyroxine to keep her euthyroid will probably be used until she reaches the age of about 18 years. Then, when she has finished school and before she goes to university or starts work, definitive treatment with radio-iodine or surgery can be used.

Sex. Antithyroid drugs are commonly used for treating women aged 20 to 40 who have developed mild Graves' disease with a normal sized gland or a small goitre, and who have a 50–60 per cent chance of having a permanent remission. However, this may not be the optimal treatment if you are contemplating starting a family in the near future. Although hyperthyroidism often reduces the frequency of menstruation and induces temporary infertility, antithyroid treatment will quickly correct this situation. Thus while having antithyroid treatment you may become pregnant. This does not present an insurmountable problem, because during pregnancy the antithyroid drug in low dosage can be given without danger to the baby inside you, and usually the treatment can be stopped 6–8 weeks before your baby is born. The block–replace regime using an antithyroid drug and thyroxine is not appropriate in pregnant women because the thyroxine does not cross the placental barrier as easily as the antithyroid drug does, and the baby is likely to be made hypothyroid. Having had the baby, you will probably need to re-start the antithyroid medication a few weeks later. The antithyroid may be secreted in your milk, but breast-feeding is not usually contraindicated, particularly if you are having propylthiouracil. Life is not made easier for you, if in addition to having to look after your new baby, you have to go to the doctor to have the treatment of your Graves' disease supervised all the time. These difficulties can largely be avoided if radio-iodine or surgery is used in young women contemplating having children, although it is customary to advise against pregnancy for 4 months after radio-iodine treatment and this treatment is best avoided unless reliable contraception (the 'pill') is used during this time.

What are the antithyroid drugs? The three most commonly used are carbimazole, methimazole, and propylthiouracil. Carbimazole and methimazole are closely related and the former is quickly converted to the latter in the body. Carbimazole is widely used in Europe and methimazole in North America. Propylthiouracil, which your doctor may call PTU, can be looked upon mainly nowadays as a second-line drug that is used if side-effects occur with one of the other two, or you become pregnant or are breast feeding.

Have these antithyroid drugs got side-effects? Yes, but they are not common, occurring in approximately 3 of every 1000 patients. Nevertheless if you are prescribed an antithyroid drug it is important that you know about the possible side-effects. They usually occur, if they are going to occur at all, during the first 2 months of treatment. In order of frequency, carbimazole or methimazole may cause nausea or mild indigestion and skin rashes. Next, and less common, may come the unusual combination of pain in the joints, a low-grade fever, and sometimes swelling of the lymphatic glands. These reactions disappear quickly when the drug is stopped and may not recur if propylthiouracil is used as an alternative.

The most serious side-effect of any of these three preparations is reduction in the white corpuscles in your blood. For unknown reasons—and fortunately it is very rare, occurring in approximately 3 per 10 000 users per year— the antithyroid drug may prevent the bone marrow making a particular type of white corpuscle, the granulocyte or neutrophil, and the number of these cells may fall, causing neutropenia, or the neutrophils may disappear from the blood almost completely, causing agranulocytosis. Neutrophils or polymorphs are essential for fighting off any microorganisms that may invade your body. Usually the first manifestation of neutropenia or agranulocytosis is a sore throat. If you are taking an antithyroid drug and develop a nasty sore throat, it is essential for you to stop taking the tablets immediately and within 24 hours you should see your doctor, or go to the hospital where you are being treated, so that a white corpuscle count can be done. If this shows that the neutrophils (granulocytes) are depleted, penicillin is usually given to kill off any possible invading organisms until such time as your bone marrow has recovered and the white corpuscles have returned to your bloodstream in normal numbers. If you are sensitive to penicillin, some other appropriate antibiotic can be used. Because agranulocytosis develops rapidly, routine measurement of the white cell count is usually not helpful in predicting its occurrence.

Radio-iodine treatment

In many respects radio-iodine is very convenient treatment for Graves' disease, although it takes about 2 months to be fully effective. For reasons given in Chapter 6, radio-iodine is probably best avoided if you have bad ophthalmopathy. The advantages of radio-iodine are:

- you take it by mouth in the form of a capsule or a number of capsules or, alternatively, as a drink which you suck through a straw;

- you do not usually have to be admitted to hospital;

- you avoid, as compared with surgery, an anaesthetic, the pain of an operation and a scar on your neck and most of the potential complications;

- you are only off work for about a week or a little longer, depending upon the dose you are given;

- it is cheaper than surgery and is painless.

Radio-iodine has been used for the treatment of Graves' disease for 50 years and has proved itself safe. There has been no adverse effects from the irradiation, such as the later development of leukaemia, no lack of fertility, and no genetic abnormalities in subsequent offspring. Nevertheless, it is not given if you are pregnant because from the third month of pregnancy the thyroid gland of your baby takes up iodine and hence its thyroid would be irradiated too. Nor is radio-iodine usually used for the treatment of patients less than 15 years old unless there is some special reason.

What then are the disadvantages? You may have slight soreness of the neck for a few days. Then there is the inconvenience that after you have been given your dose of radio-iodine you are radioactive. Most of this radioactivity will be eliminated in your urine within a week. During this time you should not kiss anyone and you should not get closer than 1 metre to babies or children. Nor should you be in close proximity to other adults, whose exposure depends on how long you are with them, how close you get to them, and what dose you have been given.

Another surmountable disadvantage is that although radio-iodine has some early effect on the making of T_4 and T_3 by your thyroid cells, its maximum effect is not apparent for about 2 or 3 months. In other words, its action is slower than that of antithyroid drugs, which produce a noticeable improvement in a week or two. While waiting for the radio-iodine to work, you can be kept comfortable from the symptomatic point-of-view with a beta-blocker, such as propranolol. In severe cases of thyrotoxicosis, antithyroid drugs are given before and after the radio-iodine and continued until the ^{131}I has produced its maximum beneficial effect.

The main disadvantage of radio-iodine, which must be weighed against its many advantages, is the liability for the thyroid gland to become underactive in the ensuing years. Over a period of 2–20 years after ^{131}I treatment more than 80 per cent of patients with Graves' disease become hypothyroid. The incidence of thyroid deficiency is not materially influenced by the dose of radio-iodine given, although the larger the dose the earlier the underactivity is likely to come on.

This disadvantage is less of a practical problem than you might think, although many women are understandably fearful at the prospect that they might become fat and bloated as a result of thyroid deficiency. This will not be allowed to happen. Provided you are kept under observation, the chances of you experiencing thyroid deficiency are small, because replacement therapy with thyroxine will be started as soon as your TSH level starts to rise above normal—before you notice any physical changes. Many clinics follow-up their patients who have been treated with radio-iodine by an annual postal questionnaire, with or without a blood test, but ideally you should see your doctor every year and have a TSH and free T_4 blood test done.

Judging the correct dose of radio-iodine is difficult for the doctor. If too little is given, you will remain thyrotoxic and will need a second or even third dose. If too much is given, the sooner you are likely to become hypothyroid, but with close observation this will be countered by giving you thyroxine replacement treatment. In some centres the dose is calculated by the size of the thyroid gland and its avidity in taking up a tracer dose of isotope. In others the philosophy is to accept that sooner or later after treatment you are likely to become hypothyroid and therefore why not give a sizeable dose of ^{131}I and prescribe thyroxine as soon as the TSH level rises? This has the advantage that you will not worry about becoming hypothyroid and you will not have to be followed-up so often.

Thus in accepting radio-iodine treatment for your Graves' disease you should also accept the likelihood of needing thyroxine replacement therapy in due course, although this is not inevitable.

Surgery

In skilled hands surgical removal of most of the thyroid gland is a very effective form of treatment for Graves' disease. Before the operation you must first be rendered euthyroid either with an antithyroid drug or Lugol's iodine—sometimes both. It is dangerous to operate on an unprepared still thyrotoxic patient because this might provoke a thyroid crisis (p. 153). Although some surgeons operate when the patients's symptoms have only been controlled with a beta-blocker, this is not a practice we subscribe to because you are not euthyroid even though your pulse rate may have fallen to normal and you are feeling much better. Furthermore, this effect is rapidly lost if the tablets are missed out or not taken because of nausea.

In the hands of an experienced surgeon and a skilled anaesthetist you are unlikely to be in hospital for longer than a week—usually less. Although the appearance of the scar can never be guaranteed, the incision in the skin is made across the neck in one of the natural creases already there. In most instances it eventually becomes a fine line that looks like a normal crease and the techniques of plastic surgery are used to close the wound after some seven-eighths of the gland have been removed. Most surgeons tend deliberately to remove rather too much than too little. This is to avoid leaving too much of the gland with the risk that the remnant is sufficiently large to sustain a recurrence of your hyperthyroidism. If this should happen, a second operation, although possible, is best avoided because second operations are followed by an increased risk of complications (see below). If there is a postoperative recurrence of thyrotoxicosis, radio-iodine is used in patients of any age or sex to cure the condition.

Surgical treatment is usually preferred if:

• the goitre is retrosternal;

• it is very large and cosmetically unsightly; or

• it is compressing or displacing the windpipe.

If you have pressure on the trachea you may experience some difficulty in breathing, but before this happens you may make a curious crowing noise when you are asleep, and this may alarm your partner. This stridor, as it is called, occurs as your head slumps forwards or to one side when you are fast asleep, and the relaxed neck muscles allow the enlarged thyroid gland to compress the windpipe even more.

Prolonged treatment with an antithyroid drug or radio-iodine therapy are best avoided under these circumstances because either form of treatment may temporarily increase the size of your goitre and aggravate the degree of compression.

Complications of surgery

Hypothyroidism. In about 20 per cent or more of surgically treated patients hypothyroidism develops in the first year or so postoperatively. The surgeon cannot be blamed for this because he has rightly veered towards removing too much, rather than too little, of the gland. After the operation you will be followed-up and if thyroid underactivity is going to develop as a direct consequence of the surgery this is usually apparent within 3 months. Thyroid deficiency may also develop later on because of autoimmune destruction of your thyroid cells. It is important for anyone who has had a thyroidectomy to have their T_4 and TSH measured annually. If hypothyroidism develops, it is easily treated by taking thyroxine tablets by mouth to make good the deficit.

Two other complications may follow surgery but both are extremely rare.

Trouble with your voice. Running on either side of the neck, in or near the thyroid gland, are the nerves that activate the vocal cords (the recurrent laryngeal nerves). If these are bruised at the time of the operation you may have a temporarily hoarse voice afterwards, although some huskiness is not uncommon for a day or two simply as a result of the anaesthetic. Permanent hoarseness will occur only if one of the nerves to the vocal cords is actually cut, but this seldom happens with an experienced thyroid surgeon.

Muscle cramps. The other possible postoperative complication is related to change to the parathyroid glands. Usually there are four of these pea-sized glands (two on each side) which lie towards the back of the thyroid gland, or they may be embedded in it. The surgeon makes every endeavour not to damage these parathyroid glands and it is most unusual for the blood supply to all four to be permanently cut off. But they may be bruised during the operation and therefore may not function normally for some days or weeks afterwards.

The parathyroid glands regulate the level of calcium in your blood. If they do not function properly, the level of calcium falls and this may give rise to a condition called tetany. In the unlikely event of this happening to you, the first thing you may notice is a feeling of numbness of your lips and around your mouth. Later you may experience cramp in the hands and sometimes in the feet. These symptoms are corrected by giving you calcium and vitamin D or one of its related compounds to restore your blood calcium level to normal. Usually this treatment is necessary for only a short time.

Treatment of pretibial myxoedema

The course of pretibial myxoedema is unpredictable. Almost invariably it occurs in patients who have bad eye problems (ophthalmopathy). As your hyperthyroidism responds to treatment, so the skin changes on the legs may improve. In some patients, however, pretibial myxoedema may pre-date hyperthyroidism or it may not occur until after your thyrotoxicosis has been cured.

The most effective treatment is to apply a potent corticosteroid ointment each night to the affected areas on your leg, rub it well in, and then wrap pieces of polythene film (Clingfilm, Saranwrap, Klingfilm) around the involved parts of the leg. This treatment may have to be continued for quite a long time (Fig. 11, p. 44).

A few words of comfort

Graves' disease is not an easy disease for anyone to have. You will appreciate that whether you are treated with antithyroid drugs, radio-iodine, or surgery there is no immediate or instant cure. It is upsetting to have to take antithyroid drugs for a period as long as 12–18 months. Radio-iodine may not produce its maximum effect for 3 months or more. If you elect to have surgery, it will be necessary for you to be prepared for this because you must be rendered euthyroid before the operation is done. Even when you are better, follow-up, albeit infrequent, is necessary, usually for the rest of your life.

The emotional or psychological accompaniments of Graves' disease are very real. Do not blame yourself if you are unduly anxious or find yourself irritable. This problem will pass, but you must be patient.

Matters are made worse if you suffer from the eye complications of Graves' disease (Chapter 5). These can be more worrying to a woman than any other aspect of the condition. Here, too, you must try to be patient. There are special treatments for ophthalmopathy (p. 69). Later surgery may greatly improve the appearance of your eyes, but this is usually not done until the thyroid overactivity has been cured.

Questions and Answers

Q.1.   It doesn't mean I have cancer if my Graves' disease is treated with radio-iodine, does it?

A.   Graves' disease is not a malignant or cancerous condition. The answer is absolutely no.

Q.2.   I have four children. Will they also get thyroid overactivity?

A.   Not necessarily, but there is a chance that one or other of them could develop some auto-immune thyroid disease—either Graves' disease or Hashimoto's thyroiditis—later in life (see Chapters 7 and 15).

Q.3   Will I get fat after I'm treated?

A.   If you've lost weight, you will probably regain it. If you were not fat originally, there is no reason for you to become fat after you've been treated for thyroid overactivity.

Q.4   Will radio-iodine have any effect on any babies I have later on?

A.   No. Nor will it affect your fertility.

Q.5   I can feel my heart pounding away at night, and sometimes this keeps me awake. Can anything be done to stop this?

A.   Certainly. Treatment with a beta-blocker will probably help you until your overactive thyroid gland has been brought under control.

Q.6   I used to love hot weather but now I can't stand it. We've booked a family holiday in Spain this August. Should we cancel it?

A.   It is now April, and by August you should be euthyroid. By then you will not mind the lovely weather in Spain. No, don't cancel your holiday.

Q.7   I'm very short-tempered with the kids and snap at my husband all the time. Can you give me anything to stop this? Usually I'm a pretty tolerant, even-tempered sort of person.

A.   Yes, we can give a beta-blocker for a while but as your thyroid condition improves you will stop being so irritable and edgy.

Q.8   Won't surgery leave a nasty scar?

A.   Almost certainly not. Usually it gradually fades to become like another crease in your neck.

Q.9   Which of the various treatments would you recommend me to have for my Graves' disease, doctor? I am 25 years old and hope to marry next year.

A.   This depends so much upon your particular circumstances and the advantages and disadvantages of the three treatments we've already discussed. Let me draw up for you a summary of the different treatments, the procedures, and their complications:

Table A Choice of treatments for Graves' disease

Treatment	Procedure	Disadvantages	Cost
Subtotal thyroidectomy if experienced surgeon available	Once and for all treatment. Two weeks' preparation with an antithyroid drug and Lugol's iodine. Five days in hospital. One week's convalescence. Two six-weekly follow-up visits. Annual review	No surgery is pleasant. Post operative discomfort. A scar. Postoperative complications are rare except for hypothyroidism	Highest
Radio-iodine	Usually out-patient treatment. Off work 1–2 weeks. Two or three follow-up visits over a year. Annual review	Liable to hypothyroidism. Not suitable if pregnancy contemplated in the next 6 months	Lowest
Antithyroid drug	Treatment for a minimum of a year with regular visits to GP or hospital	No guarantee of a cure. About 50% of patients relapsed. Problems if starting a family	Intermediate

5
The eye changes associated with Graves' disease

The eye changes in thyroid overactivity generally

Certain eye changes are common in thyroid overactivity irrespective of its cause but fortunately in most hyperthyroid patients these are not too troublesome, although they may cause you concern. Two distinct types of ophthalmic disorder may occur. One type is due to overactivity of the sympathetic nervous system and may occur in hyperthyroidism of any cause. The other type occurs only in autoimmune hyperthyroidism.

There is likely to be a tendency for your upper eyelids to be pulled upwards, exposing more of the white of your eyes. Thus you may notice, or your relatives or friends may comment, that your eyes have developed a staring quality, like that of an actress when she wishes to convey an impression of anxiety or terror. This is called lid retraction (Fig. 10, p. 44). When you look down, the upper lids may be slow to follow the downward movement of your eyeballs—a condition called lid lag (Fig. 12). These changes may occur in hyperthyroidism due to any cause and get better as the thyroid overactivity is brought under control.

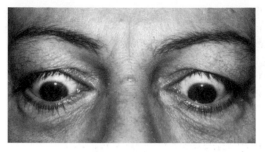

Figure 12 Lid lag. As the patient looks downwards, the upper lid lags behind the eyeball.

Eye changes peculiar to autoimmune hyperthyroidism (Graves' disease)

More troublesome are the eye changes that may occur only in Graves' disease and also, but very seldom, in Hashimoto's thyroiditis. The relationship in time between the thyroid disease and the involvement of the eyes varies. Usually the eye changes occur simultaneously with the onset of your thyroid overactivity but sometimes they precede it by several weeks or months. Less often the eyes may go wrong months or even years after your thyroid overactivity has been treated and cured.

When associated with thyroid disease—past, present, or future—the condition is known as dysthyroid eye disease or Graves' ophthalmopathy. However, sometimes the eye changes occur before or even without there ever being any overactivity of the thyroid gland at all, and this condition is called ophthalmic Graves' disease.

The changes usually affect both eyes, but sometimes only one eye is involved, or one eye may be worse than the other.

What causes the eye changes in Graves' disease?

There is inflammation of the tissues surrounding your eyeballs which lie in rigid bony sockets in your skull. The cause of this inflammation is an autoimmune reaction, mainly directed at the muscles that move your eyes from side to side and up and down (the oculomotor muscles). The anti-bodies that cause the inflammatory response are not exactly the same as those that stimulate your thyroid gland because the eye changes may occur independently of changes in thyroid function.

What may happen to your eyes?

The inflammation causes swelling of the tissues around and behind the eyeballs and increases the pressure in the rigid bony orbits. This leads to a number of problems which may occur separately or together, and do not progress in any pre-dictable manner.

1. Your eyes may be pushed forwards; this is known as prop-tosis or exophthalmos. This makes them more prominent and staring (Fig. 13). Your hospital doctor may measure

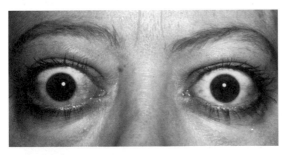

Figure 13 Exophthalmos or proptosis. Both eyeballs are more prominent than normal and protrude forwards. There is some swelling of the soft tissues above the upper eyelids. Note also that the eyes are somewhat bloodshot, the right more than the left.

painlessly how far your eyes are pushed forward with an instrument called an exophthalmometer (Fig. 14).

2. The increased pressure in the orbits may impair the normal drainage of fluid from your eyes so that your

upper eyelids become puffy and even more swollen if there is involvement of the glands above the eyes that form tears (Fig. 15). Impaired drainage from your lower lids may lead to 'bags' forming under your eyes.

3. Because your eyes are pushed forward they are less protected by the eyelids and therefore more exposed to

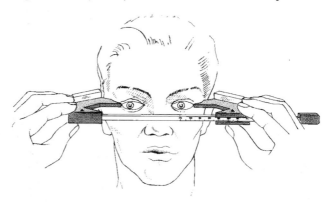

Figure 14 An exophthalmometer being used to measure the degree of protrusion of the eyes.

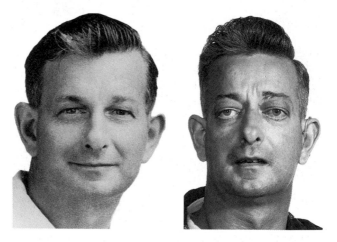

Figure 15 Appearance before (left) and after (right) the development of thyrotoxicosis.

irritation from dust, wind, and infection. You may have a feeling of grittiness or soreness in your eyes which water a lot so that almost unconsciously you keep dabbing your eyes with your handkerchief. The outer membrane covering your eyes may become inflamed and this increases the discomfort. Often the eyes appear as if they were water-logged and they may become bloodshot at the outer corners (Fig. 16, below). In the earliest phases, if there are no features of hyperthyroidism, the appearance of your eyes may be mistaken for conjunctivitis.

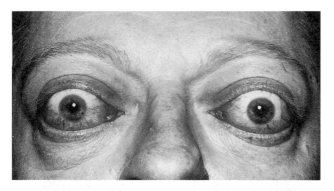

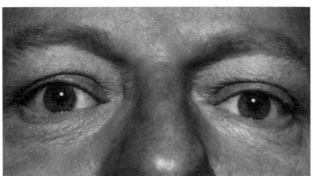

Figure 16 (a) Marked ophthalmopathy showing exophthalmos, lid retraction, and increased redness. (b) The same patient after 2 years' treatment, including decompression of both orbits.

4. The muscles that move your eyeballs in different directions may be affected so that the eyes cease to move as well as they normally do (ophthalmoplegia). Usually upward gaze is first affected and you may discover that you cannot look up without tilting your head back, which may explain the aching discomfort in the back of your neck. Later, movement of your eyes from side to side may be impaired. Because the eyeballs no longer move exactly in parallel with each other you may develop double vision (diplopia). When looking straight ahead you will see a pencil held up straight in front of you by your doctor as one. When, however, he moves the pencil upwards or to one side you see two pencils.

5. The increased pressure in your bony orbits may affect the optic nerves that carry the visual image from your eyes to the brain. This may threaten your eyesight.

Severe ophthalmopathy which may affect your vision is sometimes called 'malignant exophthalmos' (Fig. 17, p. 71). This is not a good term because the condition has nothing to do with cancer. Nevertheless it emphasizes the seriousness of the condition which, unless treated, could lead to blindness.

How does the doctor know what is wrong?

The cause of the eye changes is usually obvious when your doctor finds you are thyrotoxic, but the diagnosis may be more difficult if you do not have thyroid overactivity and particularly if the changes involve only one eye, because other disorders in the orbit may produce the same appearances. The presence of thyroid autoantibodies in your blood favours ophthalmic Graves' disease and about 60 per cent of people with this condition have thyroid peroxidase antibodies and 90 per cent or more have thyroid-stimulating antibodies. Furthermore, the TSH level is often below the reference range despite the level of the thyroid hormones not yet being raised in ophthalmic Graves' disease before hyperthyroidism develops.

Special X-rays or ultrasound examination of the orbits may be needed to confirm the diagnosis. Computer-assisted tomography (a CT or CAT scan) or an MRI scan shows what is going on in the orbits by taking multiple sliced pictures of your eye sockets. In ophthalmopathy there is a characteristic thickening of the oculomotor muscles (Fig. 8, p. 35).

It is likely that you will have to see a specialist eye doctor who may carry out any one of a number of tests to:

- assess whether your general eyesight is all right;
- be sure that your ability to see different colours is normal;
- be sure that the membranes covering your eyeball are not damaged;
- measure the pressure in your eyeballs;
- see whether your fields of vision are normal; and
- chart the movements of your eyes to see that the eyeballs are moving properly in all directions and in parallel.

Treatment

For unknown reasons, the eye changes are often worse in those who smoke cigarettes and in the older man, but if your eye problems are mild and do not get worse, you will probably not need any special treatment for them.

In two-thirds of patients the stariness of the eyes caused by lid retraction diminishes as their thyroid overactivity is brought under control. The elevation of the upper lids may also be reduced by treatment with a beta-blocker. If the lid retraction and lid lag persist, surgery to lower the position of the eyelids has a strikingly beneficial effect.

There is evidence that treatment of the thyroid overactivity in Graves' disease with radio-iodine may aggravate the eye changes more than does treatment with an antithyroid drug. Although this has not been proven conclusively, many doctors believe it prudent to treat the Graves' disease medically to start with and see what effect this has on your eyes. If radio-iodine is used in patients with mild or moderate ophthalmopathy, it is usually wise to cover this under the protection of corticosteroids. It is important to avoid making you thyroid deficient because this, too, may aggravate your eye problems.

When the eyes are swollen and feel gritty, methyl cellulose eye-drops by day and a lubricating ointment at night often help. You may find that your eyes are less puffy if you sleep propped up with several pillows. Sometimes the temporary use of a diuretic tablet that increases the elimination of fluid from the body helps. Your eyes may be more comfortable if you wear dark glasses with side pieces to protect them from the wind and dust.

Double vision tends to improve in two-thirds of patients when their thyroid overactivity is brought under control. Persistent double vision, however, is a great nuisance and handicap. During the early phases you may find that reading or watching television is made more tolerable by wearing a patch over one eye. If you wear spectacles, painting clear nail varnish over the inside of one lens will mean that you see only one image. Alternatively, special prisms can be supplied or fitted to your existing spectacles to correct the double vision and allow you to drive safely. Later when the condition of the eyes has become static, an eye surgeon may correct the muscle imbalance so that the double vision is permanently cured or at least much improved.

A reduction in the protrusion of the eyes occurs spontaneously, but slowly, in about 20 per cent of patients as the thyroid overactivity is controlled. In more than half the patients it remains static and in about 20 per cent it becomes worse unless special treatment is given.

To reduce the protrusion of your eyes corticosteroids (prednisone or methylprednisolone), which are akin to cortisone, can be effective, as shown in Fig. 17, and may be used in conjunction with other drugs that suppress the

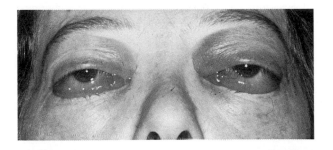

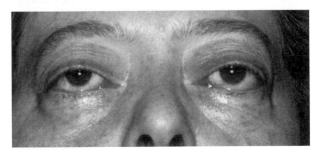

Figure 17 (a) Severe ophthalmopathy in Graves' disease before treatment. The eyeballs are protruding forwards but the extent of this exophthalmos is in part masked by the swelling in and around the eyelids. (b) Ten days after treatment with prednisone (a corticosteroid drug) the ophthalmopathy is much improved. The eyes are less 'angry' and uncomfortable. The swelling of the eyelids is much reduced, but upward movement of the eyeballs is still defective, which explains why the patient holds her head tilted back.

autoimmune reaction going on in your orbits. Sometimes you may be advised to have the outer part of your eyelids sewn together under a local anaesthetic because by narrowing the opening between the eyelids, better coverage and protection of your eyeballs is obtained and the cosmetic appearance is improved. In severe cases deep X-ray therapy to the orbits is very effective but this treatment must be given by an experienced radiotherapist who will protect the lenses of your eyes from irradiation that could cause cataracts to develop later.

Rarely, in less than 10 per cent of patients, is it necessary to protect the optic nerves and prevent blindness by enlarging the bony orbits to allow the swollen tissue behind the eyeballs to expand and thus reduce the pressure. Various surgical operations to achieve this have been devised. Nowadays usually the floor of the bony orbit is removed from inside the mouth without making any visible external scar. The improvement from ocular discomfort, threatened vision, and in the appearance of the eyes can be striking (Fig. 16, p. 67).

The eye changes that may occur in Graves' disease are without doubt the most upsetting for any patient. The ophthalmopathy is difficult to treat and, sadly, despite the best treatments available at present, a proportion of patients may have persistent eye problems.

Questions and Answers

Q.1 Do all patients with Graves' disease get eye problems?

A. No, or only minor or temporary ones. Many thyrotoxic patients (80 per cent) have no major complaints about their eyes throughout the whole course of their illness.

Q.2 Why aren't you doing more to help me with my eye trouble?

A. Because we have not yet controlled your overactive thyroid gland and it is too early to tell which way 'the cat is going to jump'. Hopefully your eyes will improve as your thyroid comes under control and no special treatment for your eyes will be necessary.

Q.3 My eyes feel much less gritty this month and are watering less. Is this a good sign?

A. Yes, this is what we like to see happen. There is likely to be further improvement.

Q.4   I used to have nice eyes. Now they took terrible! I've got this puffiness over my upper eyelids and bags under my lower ones. What can I do about this?

A.   Sleep, if you can, propped up with more pillows. I'll give you a diuretic to increase your urine output which may also help. Try not to worry too much. When your thyroid problem has been put right, we can do something more about your eyes if they're still a problem. Surgery, if necessary, may be helpful later.

Q.5   Will my eyes get better when you've cured my hyperthyroidism?

A.   Almost certainly yes, but it will take time. The condition of your eyes is likely to fluctuate and it is too early to say what the final appearance is going to be. When you are euthyroid and everything else has settled down, we may recommend some minor surgery to improve the appearance of your eyes and this is usually very successful. For the moment we must wait and see.

6
Other causes of thyroid overactivity

Although Graves' disease is the most common cause of thyroid overactivity, you may become hyperthyroid under a number of other circumstances, which are listed below roughly in the order of their frequency, although this varies in different parts of the world.

- a toxic multinodular goitre (p. 76);
- a solitary toxic 'hot' adenoma (p. 76);
- as a result of having subacute virus thyroiditis (see Chapter 9);
- postpartum thyroiditis (silent thyroiditis) (p. 151);
- in association with Hashimoto's thyroiditis, so called Hashitoxicosis (see Chapter 7);
- as a result of taking too much thyroxine, triiodothyronine, or thyroid extract by mouth (p. 77);
- thyroid overactivity induced by taking iodine or iodine-containing substances (p. 79);
- drug induced by such medicaments as amiodarone;
- cancer of the thyroid gland or its metastases (see Chapter 12);
- pregnancy and hyperemesis gravidarum (p. 141);
- a disorder of the pituitary gland that results in excess production of thyroid-stimulating hormone and hence thyroid overactivity (p. 149); and

- a tumour of the reproductive system (male or female) which secretes a hormone that stimulates the thyroid gland (p. 80).

In any of these situations your symptoms are likely to be much the same as in Graves' disease (Chapter 4) except that the major eye changes (ophthalmopathy) peculiar to autoimmune thyroid disease do not occur.

Toxic multinodular goitre

This condition, also known as Plummer's disease after the American physician who described it in 1913, tends to arise in the older patient, aged 50–70, who for many years has had a goitre which has gradually become larger and lumpy or nodular. The symptoms of thyrotoxicosis develop insidiously and resemble those of Graves' disease. Because of the patient's age, heart failure may be the presenting feature. An isotope scan shows that some nodules are over-active ('hot') and separated by areas of inactivity. In most patients, particularly the older ones, radio-iodine is the preferred treatment and the gland is likely to shrink in size. Pretreatment with an antithyroid drug, before the radio-iodine is given, is advisable in many patients. Surgical removal, after due preoperative preparation, is an alternative method of treatment (p. 57).

A solitary toxic 'hot' adenoma

In this condition a clump of cells, a nodule or benign tumour (an adenoma), becomes overactive and in effect takes over the function of the whole gland. The result is that all the activity is located in one area, and the rest of the gland goes into a resting state because, through the feedback mechanism, the secretion of TSH from the pituitary is switched off by the hormone output from the 'hot' nodule. The offending solitary adenoma can usually be felt by your doctor, but not always. The rest of the thyroid may not be enlarged, and indeed may be smaller than normal. The condition is most commonly seen in middle-aged and older women. In its early stages the adenoma may not produce an excess of thyroid hormones but gradually over a period of years the levels of T_4 and particularly T_3 are likely to rise and the TSH is suppressed. The key to the diagnosis is a radio-isotope scan which shows uptake in the solitary nodule (Fig. 5, p. 30), which is therefore 'hot', and there is little or no uptake by the rest of the gland.

Antithyroid drugs are effective but do not induce a permanent remission of the thyrotoxic symptoms. You can have the 'hot' nodule removed surgically but probably the best treatment is a fairly large dose of radio-iodine. This destroys the 'hot' adenoma, and the remaining normal, but previously suppressed, gland gradually resumes its normal function.

Taking too much thyroxine or triiodothyronine

For a number of reasons, people may take too much thyroxine, triiodothyronine, or sometimes thyroid extract, although the last is seldom used nowadays because it is an impure substance of variable potency. The thyroid hormone levels in your blood depend upon which of these drugs you are taking in excess. If you are taking too much thyroxine, the T_4 and probably the T_3 levels will be raised. If you are taking too much triiodothyronine, the T_3 level will be raised and the T_4 is low. Irrespective of which compound you are taking to excess, the TSH level will be low or undetectable.

Treatment of thyroid deficiency

If your thyroid is underactive, too much thyroxine (or sometimes triiodothyronine) may be prescribed while your doctor is adjusting the replacement dosage. How the correct dosage is arrived at is discussed on p. 99.

Self-treatment

Some people like being hyperthyroid; it gives them a 'high' and they treat themselves with thyroid hormones.

Sometimes they deny that they are doing this ('thyrotoxicosis factitia').

Obesity

Thyroid hormones are sometimes given to help people lose weight, but this not usually beneficial. If the dose is small, all that happens is that by the feedback mechanism the output of TSH is reduced. The thyroid gland then puts out less hormone but the level of thyroid hormones in the bloodstream remains normal because of the hormone being taken by mouth. If the dosage is larger, then the thyroid hormone levels will rise; you will become hyperthyroid and this will have an adverse effect on your heart and on your bones (osteoporosis).

In the past people were sometimes told that they were obese because they were suffering from thyroid deficiency and ever since they have taken thyroid hormones for many years. Usually the initial diagnosis was based on the results of the only tests available in those days, which were unreliable. The most sensitive test for confirming thyroid underactivity is to measure the TSH (p. 18)—a test that only became available some 20–25 years ago. Belief that the initial diagnosis was correct may have been heightened by you losing a few pounds of weight after starting the treatment. This happened because thyroid hormones promote the loss of fluid from the body, and it was the loss of water rather than of fat that was responsible for your initial weight reduction. Any further weight loss was probably more due to you eating less rather than to the thyroid hormone you were taking. It is important to emphasize that hypothyroidism is rarely the sole cause of obesity.

If you have been taking thyroxine for many years, it is important to know whether you really need this treatment, and if you do, it may be necessary to adjust the dosage because as you grow older your thyroid deficiency may well become greater. Hence it is in your best interests if your doctor advises you to stop taking the hormone for

6–8 weeks and then have a modern sensitive test done (measurement of your TSH level) to decide whether you really need it.

Iodine-containing substances

Contrast substances ('dyes') used in special X-ray procedures and some 'health' foods, such as Kelp, which is made from seaweed, contain a lot of iodine which may induce thyroid overactivity in susceptible individuals.

In some instances the thyroid overactivity remits if the increased intake of iodine is stopped, and until this happens your symptoms can usually be controlled with a beta-blocker. In other people the hyperthyroidism persists and the condition is treated in the same way as Graves' disease or a toxic multinodular goitre.

Drug-induced hyperthyroidism

Drugs, such as amiodarone which is useful for controlling certain irregular heart rhythms, may disturb thyroid function. Other medicaments, such as cough medicines which contain iodine, may also cause hyper- and hypothyroidism. Lithium may induce hypothyroidism.

Pregnancy and hyperemesis gravidarum

These are discussed on p. 141.

Tumours that cause thyroid overactivity

These conditions are rare, but thyroid overactivity may occur in association with a number of different types of tumour.

Cancer of the thyroid gland which usually has spread to other parts of the body may cause hyperthyroidism. The presence of these overactive cells can be shown by a whole-body radio-iodine scan and they can be killed off with radio-iodine treatment (p. 133).

A tumour of your pituitary gland that secretes excess TSH will stimulate your thyroid to increased activity. Radio-iodine or technetium uptake by your thyroid gland will be increased but the TSH level will be normal or high instead of being depressed or undetectable as it is in the much more common causes of thyroid overactivity.

A tumour of the ovary which contains thyroid-like tissue may secrete excess T_4 and/or T_3. An isotope scan of the thyroid gland will show little or no uptake whereas a scan of the offending ovary will show a high uptake.

A tumour of the testis or ovary may produce a hormone that stimulates your thyroid gland. An isotope scan will show increased uptake by your thyroid, but usually the underlying tumour in the testis or ovary will already have produced local symptoms of which your doctor must be made aware.

The treatment of all these tumorous conditions is directed at the primary underlying cause.

Questions and Answers

Q.1   What exactly is a solitary toxic nodule?
A.   It is a cluster of cells that have taken over the func-
      tion of the rest of your thyroid gland. These cells are
      now producing too much thyroid hormones, which
      is why you feel as you do.

Q.2   So I have a toxic nodule. I haven't got cancer then?
A.   Certainly not.

Q.3   But I've been taking thyroxine 300 micrograms for
      20 years—ever since my thyroid operation. Are you
      telling me to stop after all this time?

A.   300 micrograms is a large dose. You probably don't need so much. I can say that because your TSH level is depressed and the free thyroxine level in your blood is way up above normal. This is not good for your heart nor for your bones, which may be getting thinner now anyway because you are having the change of life. I think we may find that 200 micrograms is perfectly adequate for you.

Q.4   But I thought iodine was good for you. That's why I'm taking Kelp; lots of my friends do too.

A.   Certainly iodine is good for anyone. We all need *some* iodine but not too much. In your case your thyroid gland has become overactive.

Q.   Will it stop being overactive when I stop taking Kelp?

A.   We can't be sure. It may or it may not. We shall just have to see. Even if you remain thyrotoxic, we can always put that right.

Q.5   You say I have an enlarged thyroid gland which is overactive and contains many nodules. I feel pretty well but the swelling is very unsightly and getting bigger I think. What can you do about the swelling? Cosmetically it's not very nice, you know.

A.   I quite agree. Radio-iodine treatment will stop the gland being overactive and in a year's time will have reduced its size very significantly.

7
Hashimoto's thyroiditis

Hashimoto's thyroiditis—also known as chronic lymph-adenoid or lymphocytic goitre—is an important and common disease. It is called after the Japanese surgeon who first described it in 1912, but the condition was not properly understood until British doctors discovered thyroid autoantibodies in 1956.

- It affects about 1 in 10 women aged 30 years or over.

- It is an important cause of goitre, especially in women, but may also affect female children and adolescents.

- It affects women 10 times more often than men.

- It is an important cause of thyroid underactivity (hypothyroidism). In many parts of the Western world it is the most common cause of thyroid deficiency, although lack of iodine ranks first world-wide.

- Over the years a goitre caused by Hashimoto's thyroiditis may disappear and the thyroid gland is replaced by fibrous tissue (atrophic hypothyroidism).

Cause of Hashimoto's thyroiditis

As explained in Chapter 2, Hashimoto's thyroiditis is an autoimmune disorder and is caused by the presence of certain antibodies that react with the cells of the thyroid gland. Why these antibodies arise is not understood, but they develop more commonly in people with a particular genetic make-up and thus there is often a history of thyroid or other autoimmune diseases in the person's immediate family or distant relatives (see Chapter 15). The so-called microsomal or thyroid peroxidase (TPO) and thyroglobulin antibodies that appear in the blood and are formed by certain white corpuscles (lymphocytes), invade the thyroid gland and slowly destroy the thyroid cells.

Course of Hashimoto's thyroiditis

The course of the disease is protracted over many years, and during this time may wax and wane in its destructive effect on the thyroid gland. At any stage the progression of the disease may appear to be arrested and to lie dormant. If you develop Hashimoto's thyroiditis, you may become aware of it and seek medical advice at many different stages along the road. For example, the development of a small goitre, usually painless but sometimes associated with mild discomfort, may be in you the first manifestation of the disease. The goitre often feels rubbery and slightly knobbly. Alternatively and perhaps more commonly, you may not be aware that anything is wrong until later in the course of the condition when you become thyroid deficient.

A small proportion of people with Hashimoto's thyroiditis experience, usually early in the course of the disease, mild symptoms of thyroid overactivity—so-called Hashitoxicosis—for a few weeks or months. If you experience this, you will have the symptoms of Graves' disease and you may even have some of the eye changes of that condition (Chapters 4 and 5). Hashitoxicosis is due to thyroid-stimulating antibodies enhancing thyroid activity but the hyperthyroidism seldom lasts long because the thyroid destructive antibodies are more dominant.

What do you feel?

In the early stages of Hashimoto's disease you will feel perfectly well but you or your family may notice that you have a small, painless goitre. Rarely you may experience some slight discomfort in the front of your neck or tenderness on pressure. For a period of a month or two, often intermittently, you may have slight discomfort or be consciousness of a swelling in your neck when you swallow.

If you are one of the few people who have a temporary period of Hashitoxicosis, you will feel ill, loose weight, have pounding of your heart, feel overheated, and be intolerant of hot weather. You may have looseness of your bowels, and your eyes may become starey. Indeed, you may have any or all of the symptoms and signs of Graves' disease (Chapters 4 and 5). Later in the course of the disease, as your thyroid gland functions less adequately, you will develop the symptoms of thyroid deficiency (Chapter 8) but these may be wrongly attributed to the menopause or simply to you growing older.

How is the diagnosis confirmed?

Essentially the diagnosis of Hashimoto's thyroiditis is based on finding thyroid peroxidase (TPO) antibodies in your blood. The level of these often increases as the disease progresses. In the late stages if the thyroid gland is destroyed and becomes atrophic, no thyroid tissue will be left and the level of these autoantibodies may fall to low or undetectable levels.

The function of the thyroid gland has to be monitored at intervals throughout the long course of Hashimoto's thyroiditis despite you experiencing few, if any symptoms, beyond having a small goitre. Although treatment with thyroxine often prevents your goitre from becoming larger or may reduce its size, this therapy becomes essential when the T_4 level begins to fall. There has been debate as to whether treatment with thyroxine should be started before obvious overt hypothyroidism has appeared, when only the TSH level is raised and the free T_4 level is normal (Chapter 8, Table 3, p. 92). Some doctors find it logical to start treatment with thyroxine when there is evidence of impending thyroid failure as shown by a normal T_4 level but an unquestionably raised TSH with the presence of thyroid autoantibodies, because about 5 per cent per annum of such women with only a raised TSH level become overtly hypothyroid and develop a low T_4. No harm comes from starting treatment early and you may find that you feel considerably better because with hindsight you realize that you have been suffering from mild ill-health that crept up on you so silently that you did not notice it.

Not only must Hashimoto's thyroiditis be diagnosed but you and your doctor should be aware that it is possible that you may also develop one of the other autoimmune diseases (Chapter 15).

Treatment

We have no safe reliable way of modifying the faulty immunological system that mistakenly believes your thyroid cells are 'foreign'. Thus the basic cause of Hashimoto's thyroiditis is untreatable, although the symptoms can be totally alleviated.

If you have a temporary phase of Hashitoxicosis, a beta-blocker and/or antithyroid medication, such as carbimazole, may be given for a short time (p. 50). If the gland becomes uncomfortably painful, a short course of corticosteroids may be used, as in subacute viral thyroiditis (p. 108).

In general, the treatment is replacement therapy for the thyroid failure, although a goitre may sometimes be prevented from becoming larger or even reduced in size by giving thyroxine. The essential step is the prevention of hypothyroidism when this is imminent or the correction of hypothyroidism when it has developed. The best treatment is replacement therapy with thyroxine (p. 99).

Occasionally surgery is required, particularly if there is any possibility that the goitre is due to cancer and not to Hashimoto's disease. This difficulty may arise when the thyroid feels very hard or is enlarged unevenly, but usually a needle biopsy will resolve this diagnostic problem. Surgery is also advisable if you develop hoarseness of the voice, symptoms due to compression of the windpipe, or if the goitre is cosmetically unsightly despite treatment with thyroxine.

Let us follow Angela along the road of Hashimoto's disease, not forgetting that she started the condition long before we knew as much about it as we do now.

I'm now aged 60 and feel perfectly well. I take two thyroxine tablets every day—one of 0.1 mg strength and the other of 0.05 mg strength. When I was aged about 17, my mother noticed my thyroid gland was a bit big. She knew about the thyroid gland because my auntie, her sister, had Graves' disease. Over the next few years my goitre became more obvious. Our family doctor said my thyroid felt rubbery and fleshy, and I hadn't got Graves' disease. He sent me to the hospital where they found I had antibodies in my blood, but my protein-bound iodine—an old test of thyroid function they don't do any more—was normal. I felt perfectly well and the goitre didn't bother me.

At the age of 28 the goitre had become smaller but for the first time I had some discomfort in the front of my neck; it wasn't much although on a few occasions it hurt to swallow. Our doctor said my thyroid felt firmer and it was slightly tender when he pressed it.

At the age of 48 I began to feel tired. I thought it was the 'change' and having to look after my two teenage daughters. My periods were a bit heavier and I had to push myself to do the housework and the shopping. Eventually I went back to the doctor. He did some tests and said my thyroid was having difficulty in making hormone because my TSH was up and the thyroid hormone was down. Our GP said he couldn't feel my goitre any more and I was hypothyroid. That's when he started me on thyroxine. My periods came back and I didn't have the 'change' until I was 54.

Few people with Hashimoto's thyroiditis will be aware of all these different stages and not many doctors may be in practice long enough to follow an individual patient over the 30–40 years involved.

Questions and Answers

Q.1   What do you mean when you say I have an auto-immune disease?

A.   Certain defensive cells in your body that are there to fight diseases, particularly infectious diseases, have mistakenly decided that your thyroid cells are not yours—they are 'foreign' enemy cells. Hence the defensive white corpuscles are producing antibodies and these are quietly destroying your thyroid gland.

Q.2   I don't understand why I've got an underactive thyroid gland when my aunt says she had an overactive one.

A.   Both you and your aunt have related autoimmune diseases. In her case her 'soldiers', which we call antibodies, stimulated her thyroid gland whereas your antibodies are killing off your thyroid cells.

Q.3   Will the swelling in my neck get smaller with treatment?

A.   Not necessarily but it may if you take your tablets regularly and go on taking them.

Q.4   Ought I to have my children tested to see if they are going to get an autoimmune disease?

A.   At the ages of five and three they're too young. They *may* possibly develop an autoimmune disease later in life, but it is too early to tell. In other words the tests might be negative now, only to become positive later in life. It's unlikely that they will, but the best thing to do is to wait. If either of them develops a goitre, then obviously tests must be done.

8
Underactivity of the thyroid and its causes

Causes

There are many causes for thyroid deficiency in the adult. World-wide the most common is probably lack of dietary iodine (p. 4). Deficiency of this essential element precludes the thyroid cells from getting enough raw material to make sufficient hormones. This is an example of trying to make bricks without straw and is usually associated with the development of a sizeable goitre. But, as we have seen in Chapter 7, Hashimoto's disease is the most common cause of hypothyroidism in the Western world. A significant number of people develop hypothyroidism 2 or 3 months after radio-iodine treatment (p. 54) or surgery (p. 57) for the correction of thyroid overactivity. This thyroid deficiency may be transient but, particularly after radio-iodine treatment, it is likely to become permanent, the incidence increasing as the years pass.

Other less common causes of thyroid underactivity, which in some cases may be only transient or remit when the cause is removed, include:

1. Antithyroid drugs such as methimazole or carbimazole, if given in too large a dose over too long a period of time, will induce thyroid deficiency by impeding the manufacture of thyroid hormones by the thyroid cells.

2. Temporary underactivity of the gland caused by silent thyroiditis which occurs in about 1 in 10 women after

childbirth (p. 152). It may also occur transiently after viral thyroiditis (p. 109).

3. Medicines purchased over the chemist's counter, particularly for coughs, may contain iodides and in some people their prolonged usage causes underactivity of the thyroid.

4. Other medicines prescribed by doctors may interfere with the function of the thyroid gland. Lithium which is used for certain mental disorders is one such, and amiodarone used for stopping irregularity of the heart beat is another.

5. Certain foods such as cabbage and other 'greens' related to kale (notably in Tasmania), seaweed (particularly in Japan), and certain so-called health foods contain antithyroid compounds, as do some contaminated sources of water in the Third World.

6. A congenital abnormality of the chemical processes in the thyroid gland which prevents it making T_4 and T_3 properly (p. 116).

7. Sometimes thyroid failure occurs secondary to disorders that stop the pituitary gland from secreting the thyroid-stimulating hormone (TSH). Usually other hormones normally formed by the pituitary are also deficient in hypopituitarism. A major finding in this situation is a low or absent level of TSH in the blood as compared with the raised level found when the problem is confined solely to the thyroid gland.

What happens if you have an underactive thyroid gland?

Hypothyroidism is the name given to the clinical condition that develops when there is inadequate secretion of thyroxine (T_4) and to a lesser extent of triiodothyronine (T_3). Irrespective of the cause for the thyroid underactivity the symptoms are in general the same, and their severity depends upon the degree of thyroid failure and upon its duration. Myxoedema is the word used to describe untreated hypothyroidism of advanced degree and of long standing, and was originally coined to describe the thickened, cold skin often found in this state.

Hypothyroidism should be looked upon as a graded phenomenon ranging from a slight impairment of thyroid function as shown by a rise in the TSH level and few if any symptoms, and progressing through a greater reduction of thyroid hormones with more likelihood of symptoms, to complete thyroid failure that will make you feel really ill and is often obvious to your doctor and associated with very abnormal laboratory tests (Table 3).

In most instances thyroid underactivity, particularly in Hashimoto's thyroiditis, creeps up on you. The changes are so imperceptibly slow in their development that for some long time they are not recognized by you or those closest to you.

Overt hypothyroidism in the adult

The first thing you may notice is tiredness which gets progressively worse. You feel rundown and sluggish. You may find that you feel the cold more than those around you. You may want more domestic heating later in the spring or earlier in the autumn than others in your household. Unconsciously you may wear thicker clothes when the rest of the family are more lightly clad.

Your periods may become heavier and last longer; less often they stop altogether. You may gain some weight but seldom more than a few pounds. Your skin may become dry and thicker; your scalp hair may come out more than it used to. Your eyebrows may become sparse and the hair on your forearms short and stubbly. Your hands become podgy and your voice deeper in pitch. Your hearing may, unbeknown to you, become dulled so you are the last person in the house to hear the telephone ring. Your bowels are likely to be constipated (Fig. 18). Aches and cramps in the muscles are common, and in the night or on waking in the morning you may experience pins and needles in your fingers and

Table 3 The grading of thyroid failure

Grade	Symptoms of hypothyroidism	Free T$_4$	Free T$_3$	TSH
Compensated	None or non-specific	Normal	Normal	Slightly raised
Occult or mild hypothyroidism	None or mild	Slightly low	Normal	Raised
Overt hypothyroidism	Mild or marked	Low	Normal or low	Very raised

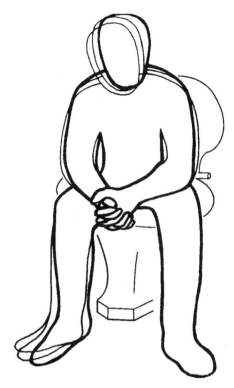

Figure 18 A representation of a patient with thyroid deficiency (hypothyroidism). The hypothyroid patient is slowed down, physically and mentally, and is likely to be constipated, as implied in this drawing. Compare with the hyperthyroid patient shown in Fig. 9 (p. 42).

hands. This is due to a nerve at the wrist becoming trapped (carpal tunnel syndrome)—a condition likely to improve when your thyroid deficiency is corrected.

The older person with thyroid deficiency may experience a tight constricting pain across the chest when walking fast or up an incline—pain which causes you to stop walking for a while until the tightness wears off. This is called angina pectoris and is due to narrowing of the coronary arteries that carry blood to your heart. Similarly if the arteries to your legs are furred up, you may experience pain in one or other calf when you walk, and this too will cause you to stop until the pain wears off (intermittent claudication).

In advanced cases of myxoedema the patient feels unsteady on her feet and once she has fallen she may be reluctant to venture out of the house alone. Words are less clearly articulated so that speech is slowed and slurred. Patients with mild hypothyroidism, and even more so those with myxoedema, may become mentally disturbed, being depressed or anxious. The patient may hear voices, believe her food is being poisoned, and become agitated. These problems will get better gradually as the thyroid deficiency is corrected. Because their metabolism is so slowed, some patients may become unconscious, particularly during cold weather, a condition known as myxoedema coma. This tends to happen in older women who live alone and are not visited by friends or relatives. Myxoedema coma seldom occurs nowadays but it is a grave condition and often ends fatally unless treated promptly in hospital.

Mild hypothyroidism

If you have a minor degree of thyroid deficiency your symptoms will be more vague. Tiredness for which you can think of no physical or emotional reason, lack of 'go', intolerance of cold, dryness of your skin, constipation, heavy periods, and a feeling of bloatedness may all occur.

What your doctor finds

Depending on the degree of thyroid deficiency and its duration, the changes in you may or may not be obvious to your doctor. If the underactivity is marked and if the doctor knows you well but has not seen you for some months, he may immediately suspect what is wrong with you. He may find that your face has become puffy. Your palms are cool and dry. Your skin may have a yellow tinge although your cheeks may remain surprisingly pink unless your heavy periods have made you anaemic. He or she may spot that your eyelids and hands are puffy, sometimes with swelling of the ankles. Your movements, your speech and thoughts may be slowed. Your heart rate is likely to be slow, and your blood pressure somewhat elevated. Your tendon reflexes are sluggish to relax (p. 24). Sometimes fluid will have collected in your abdomen, in your chest or in the pericardium (the membrane that surrounds your heart) so that you become short of breath. An electrical recording of your heart (electrocardiogram) will show characteristic changes.

If the cause of your hypothyroidism is Hashimoto's disease, your thyroid gland may be slightly enlarged, normal in size, or so destroyed that your doctor cannot feel it. If the gland can be felt, it will be harder than normal. Sometimes your doctor may find one or two nodules in it which are usually small areas of normal thyroid tissue that have escaped the autoimmune inflammatory attack of the Hashimoto's thyroiditis but are insufficient in amount to sustain normal thyroid function.

Diagnosis of adult hypothyroidism

The abnormalities in the thyroid function tests depend on the severity and duration of the deficiency (Table 3). In clinically obvious hypothyroidism, the T_4 level is depressed below the normal range and the TSH level is very high. In mild early cases the T_4 level is low normal and the TSH level is only marginally raised.

Certain indirect tests for detecting thyroid deficiency or for following its response to treatment have been used. The sluggishness of the tendon reflexes may be measured (p. 24). The blood cholesterol is often raised in thyroid deficiency and usually comes down in response to adequate treatment. The electrocardiographic changes disappear with treatment.

Your doctor is likely to look for thyroid antibodies unless he already knows that you have Hashimoto's disease or if the cause for your thyroid deficiency is obvious because you have had thyroid surgery or been treated with radio-iodine. The finding of antibodies raises the possibility that you might be subject, sooner or later, to some other auto-immune disease (p. 159).

If your doctor does not know you well, a comparison of your present appearance with an earlier photograph may be helpful in suggesting a diagnosis of hypothyroidism. Pictures taken before and after replacement treatment with thyroxine are often a witness to the striking therapeutic response (Fig. 19).

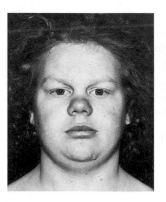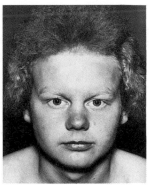

Figure 19 A 17-year-old carpenter with myxoedema (hypothyroidism): (left) before treatment; (right) after 18 months' treatment with thyroxine.

Thyroid underactivity in children

The onset of thyroid underfunction in younger children is usually due to imperfect development or maldescent (p. 2) of the thyroid gland earlier in life, or to Hashimoto's thyroiditis. Less often the cause is some congenital defect whereby the manufacture of T_4 and T_3 by the thyroid cells is impaired (dyshormonogenesis).

When the gland has not developed properly the amount of thyroid tissue may have been adequate initially to sustain normal levels of the thyroid hormones, but as the child grows the maldeveloped gland cannot keep pace and thyroid deficiency gradually develops.

The most obvious consequence of thyroid underactivity at this age is that the child stops growing. Seldom are there other symptoms and surprisingly the child's performance at school is usually maintained. Although failure to grow is the presenting feature, the child is often plump and may have pads of fat above the collar-bones.

The diagnosis is based on the same tests as are used for confirming thyroid underactivity in the adult. In addition, X-rays will show that the development of the bones is delayed in relation to the child's chronological age. An iso-tope scan of the neck may show the gland is abnormally small in maldevelopment, and in maldescent (p. 27) the uptake may be near the root of the tongue instead of in the normal position.

Thyroid underactivity in the new-born

Thyroid failure in the new-born, if unrecognized, can be disastrous because delay in treatment results in permanent mental deficiency (cretinism). In the Western world the most common cause of congenital hypothyroidism is maldevelopment or maldescent of the thyroid gland. The prevalence is one in 3500 births. Thus in developed coun-tries every new-born baby is screened to exclude thyroid deficiency.

In areas of the world where iodine deficiency is common (p. 4) the prevalence of neonatal hypothyroidism is high and the degree of mental defect and damage to the nervous system is great. In these cases the baby's mother usually has a goitre caused by lack of iodine and possibly to other antithyroid factors in her diet or drinking water. This type of endemic neonatal hypothyroidism can be prevented by giving the mother, before and during her pregnancies, injections of iodized oil or fortifying her salt or bread with iodides.

What does a baby with thyroid deficiency look like?

The answer is that in many cases the baby looks perfectly normal even to the trained experienced eye. That is why in so-called developed countries a screening test is done routinely on every new-born baby. When there are abnormal features, these depend upon the degree of thyroid deficiency and become more obvious as the baby grows older, but by then permanent damage to the brain may have occurred. Babies with thyroid deficiency fail to thrive. The baby does not kick vigorously and sleeps excessively. Constipation is the rule. The baby's cry may be croaky. The scalp hair may be short and coarse. Often the tummy is unduly protuberant; the navel may bulge outwards and be the site of a rupture. The tongue is unusually large and to the experienced eye the face may have a characteristic flat, bloated look. Left untreated, changes due to involvement of the brain appear—poor co-ordination, shakiness, and unsteadiness, with excessively brisk tendon reflexes.

Without doing a screening test many babies with neonatal thyroid deficiency are not diagnosed until they are 6 months old and by then the brain damage (cretinism) is irreversible. Although the physical changes will disappear with thyroxine treatment, the mental state is likely to remain permanently impaired.

Diagnosis of neonatal hypothyroidism

Every new-born baby should be screened for thyroid deficiency either at birth or, more usually, on the fifth day after birth. A needle prick will be made in your baby's heel and four spots of blood are placed on a special piece of paper. Two of these spots are analysed for TSH and the other two are used to screen for another congenital disease (phenyl-ketonuria). In babies with thyroid deficiency the TSH is substantially raised. When the level is not all that high, the test has to be repeated. Sometimes congenital thyroid deficiency is transient, and without treatment your baby would develop normal thyroid function. This is liable to happen in premature births and in babies of mothers who have been taking thyroid hormone, antithyroid drugs, or iodine-containing drugs during the pregnancy. It is safer to treat all infants showing a positive test, and when your baby is about a year old to stop the replacement treatment for a few weeks and carefully observe the T_4 and TSH levels. If the T_4 falls and the TSH rises, thyroxine can be restarted and your infant will not suffer any permanent damage from being temporarily deprived of the replacement treatment.

Treatment

The best treatment for thyroid deficiency is replacement therapy with thyroxine. Although man-made, medicinal thyroxine is chemically identical to the natural hormone secreted by the thyroid gland. Being a pure substance, the amount in each tablet made by a reputable pharmaceutical company is precise and accurate. Two strengths of tablet are widely available throughout the world—0.05 milligrams (mg), also expressed as 50 micrograms (μg or mcg), and 0.1 mg (100 μg or mcg). In some countries tablets of 0.025 mg (25 μg or mcg) are also available, and in others, such as the United States, additional strengths are also available (75, 88, 112, 125, 137, 159, 175, 200, and 300 μg). Thyroxine is a stable substance and the tablets have a long shelf-life.

The starting or initial dose of thyroxine you will be given will depend upon:

1. Your age. Elderly people are usually started on a small dose, such as 0.25 mg, so as not to upset their heart. This will be certainly be necessary if you already have some heart trouble (see below).

2. The duration of time you have been thyroid deficient. If your underactivity has only just occurred as a result, say,

of a thyroid operation, replacement with a larger initial dose, such as 0.1 or 0.15 mg is safe. If the deficiency is of longer standing, the initial dose may be 0.05 mg.

The dosage of thyroxine will be adjusted by your doctor according to how you feel and the results of laboratory tests. Adjustment of the dosage is unlikely to be made more often than at intervals of 6 weeks. There is a good deal of debate among thyroid experts about what the aim, as regards the results of the laboratory tests, should be. Most patients with thyroid deficiency feel at their best when the dosage of thyroxine raises their free thyroxine level towards the upper end of the normal range, or even a little above it. This usually reduces the thyroid stimulating hormone (TSH) level towards the bottom of the normal range or even a little below it, but not so low as to be undetectable. The ultimate dose of thyroxine you need will depend upon your degree of thyroid failure and your age. The total daily dose in an adult with no functioning thyroid tissue at all is usually 0.15–0.2 mg. Occasionally the dose may need to be 0.25 mg.

Thyroxine does not work fast. A tablet taken, for example, on a Monday will induce no biologically discernible effect in your body until the following Friday. Thus you need take your tablets only once a day. There is no point in taking them two or three times a day; indeed there may be a positive disadvantage in doing so because you are likely to forget a dose, particularly the midday one. Thus take your tablet once a day at a time when you will not forget—perhaps when you brush your teeth in the morning before breakfast.

Do not expect to feel miraculously better overnight. The longer you have had thyroid deficiency, the longer will it take for you to feel really well again—sometimes as long as 6–9 months. It takes this length of time for the changes in your tissues to be reversed.

Initial problems

Elderly patients, even with a small starting dose of thyroxine, may develop heart problems, such as palpitations, irregularity of the pulse, ankle swelling, or angina. A small dose of a beta-blocker, such as 10–20 mg propranolol twice or three times daily, will usually quell these symptoms.

Some people, particularly the older ones with long-standing thyroid deficiency, may during the early phases of replacement treatment experience the 'screws'—muscular aches and pains particularly in the thighs, arms, and back. Do not stop your medication if this happens to you. A simple pain-killing medicine will help make you feel more comfortable until this problem has passed.

Adjustment of the maintenance dose

Once your maintenance dose has been established, it is likely to remain stable for some time. However, many factors may induce the need for a change in your regular dosage and for this reason you should have an annual check-up with your GP or your hospital consultant. Do not take any thyroxine on the day when you go for your check-up and have a blood sample taken. The reason for this is that for about 4 hours after ingesting a tablet of thyroxine, the blood level of thyroxine peaks and will give a spuriously high reading.

Your replacement dosage of thyroxine may need adjustment from time to time for a number of reasons. For example, if you have Hashimoto's disease your degree of thyroid deficiency may increase over the years and necessitate an increased dose of thyroxine. In general, however, as you grow older your replacement dosage may need to be decreased. However, a number of circumstances may necessitate an increased dose. Should you becomes pregnant the dose will almost certainly need increasing (p. 142). Certain diseases of the small intestine or protracted diarrhoea may impair the absorption of thyroxine and call for an increased dose. A number of different medications which you may be given could impede the absorption of your thyroxine (Table 4).

If at any time you move or change doctors, it would be sensible to ask your original doctor for a signed document setting forth how your thyroid deficiency came to light, the results of the tests that confirmed the diagnosis, and your current replacement dosage of thyroxine. This may be useful if in the years to come when you go to a different doctor or go to live abroad. Your new doctor, who finds you well, may doubt the need for continued treatment and stop your thyroxine.

Table 4   Medication that may impede the adsorption of T_4 and invoke the need for an increase in thyroxine replacement therapy

Antacids
> Aluminium hydroxide (Alu-cap, Aludrox, Aluhyde, Andursil, Asilone, Diovol, Gastrocote, Gaviscon, Gelusil, Kolanticon, Maalox, Topal) and sucralfate (Antepsin, Carafate, Sulcrate)

Cholesterol lowering agent
> Cholestyramine (Cuemid, Quantalan, Questran)

Iron preparations
> Ferrous sulphate (Fefol, Feospan, Ferrograd, Feosol, Fesovit, Irofol, Pregnavite Forte, Slow-Fe)

Some people with thyroid deficiency like to take too much thyroxine in the mistaken hope that it will help them lose weight and because they claim to feel 'better' with a thyroxine level in the blood raised far above the upper normal range. There is no doubt that some people do get 'addicted' to thyroxine and take doses that make them hyperthyroid. This has an adverse effect on the heart and also induces thinning of the bones (osteoporosis) with an enhanced liability for you to break your hip, wrist, or the bones in your spine.

Other drugs have been used for the treatment of thyroid deficiency but have little to commend them. Thyroid extract is prepared from the dried thyroid glands of animals. It is an impure substance of variable biological potency with a short shelf-life. It is no longer listed in the British National Formulary.

Triiodothyronine (T_3) is sometimes used, but it has no advantage over thyroxine except in the treatment of myxoedema coma. Triiodothyronine has a quick, short duration of action and the tablets should not be taken in a single daily dose. If T_3 is used, the correct dosage cannot be judged by the blood level of total T_4 or free T_4 (both of which will be suppressed) but by the TSH and the total or free T_3 levels.

Treatment of thyroid deficiency in babies and children

This follows the same pattern as that in grown-ups. The current dosage recommended is 10–15 μg/kg/day, which amounts to about 50 μg thyroxine per day for a full-term baby. The dosage has to be increased as the baby grows older and is best judged by the free T_4 and TSH levels in the blood. Additional assessment of the response is made from the child's growth in height and from the maturing of the bones as judged by simple X-rays of the hand and wrist. A child given too much thyroxine is likely to become overactive, unduly excitable, and will grow faster than normal.

Questions and Answers

Q.1   I've taken the thyroxine tablets you first prescribed for me 6 weeks ago. Why am I not feeling any better?

A.   It is early days. It has taken months, probably years, for you to develop thyroid underactivity and it will take at least 4 months or more before you are completely well again. You'll be pleased to know that today I'm going to increase your dose of thyroxine.

Q.2   My son was diagnosed as having thyroid deficiency in hospital, just after he was born. Now he's a year old, and the hospital want to stop the thyroxine for the next month and do another test. Is that safe?

A.   Yes, it's safe and the only way of finding out if he really needs the thyroxine now.

Q.3   My period was very heavy again last month. Is this going to get better?

A.   Almost certainly. You have only been on thyroxine treatment for 6 weeks and it takes time for everything to return to normal in the gynaecological department. Don't worry.

Q.4   Does it matter when I take my thyroid tablets?

A.   No, you can take them at any time of the day provided you always remember to take them. I think most people are less likely to forget if they take them first thing in the morning when they brush their teeth.

Q.5   The tablets I got this month from the chemist are larger than the previous ones I had. The old ones were labelled 0.1 mg thyroxine but the new ones are 100 micrograms. I feel all right. Has the chemist made a mistake?

A.   No, 0.1 milligram is the same as 100 micrograms. Several different reputable manufacturers make thyroxine tablets and they are not all of the same size or the same strength. It is important to stress that they are the correct strength for you.

9
Subacute viral thyroiditis

This condition, also known as de Quervain's thyroiditis after the Swiss physician who first described it, is not uncommon. For every 10 patients with Graves' disease, a thyroid specialist may see only one case of viral thyroiditis. Because viral thyroiditis runs a self-limiting course, mild cases may never seek medical advice and there can be no doubt that even in more severe cases the correct diagnosis is often overlooked.

The condition occurs more commonly in women than in men. The inflammation of the thyroid is caused by one of several viruses. The most common is perhaps the Coxsackie virus (first isolated in a small township of that name in New York State) but the mumps virus and others may be the cause. Attempts are seldom made to identify the causative virus in any particular patient because this is expensive and difficult, and we do not have effective drugs against many viruses.

What is subacute viral thyroiditis like?

The disease varies from very mild to quite severe. One of the authors (R.I.S.B.), having had mild de Quervain's thyroiditis himself, is in a good position to tell you:

One summer's day, when I was aged 45, I felt exceptionally and inexplicably tired. I just felt rotten. I went to bed immediately after supper and, feeling hot, I took my temperature. I had a slight fever of 37.7 °C (99 °F). I slept all right but next morning woke with a generalized headache and ached all over. My temperature was only marginally raised so I went to work. Again, I went to bed early and the headache was bad enough for me to take an aspirin. I reckoned I'd got 'flu. The next few days were much the same. After a week of coming home early and going to bed, my wife reminded me that a professor of endocrinology from out of town was coming to dine with us. He was an old friend so I came down to supper in my dressing gown, and told him I was getting over a brief attack of 'flu.

After dinner my professor friend asked, 'Are you sure you haven't got viral thyroiditis?'

'I shouldn't think so,' I said. 'Why do you ask?'

'Because you've been gently massaging your neck all evening as though it hurt and your thyroid is a bit enlarged.'

'Well, now you mention it, it does hurt.' I prodded my thyroid gland. 'Yes, it's quite tender and it hurts a bit when I swallow too. What's more I get stabs of pain that run up the side of my neck to just under my ears.'

The next day I was worse and asked our family doctor, who lives close by and was a good friend, to look in. He took my history and examined me from top to toe. (I did not mention thyroiditis because doctors who make a self-diagnosis can also make fools of themselves!) The GP looked puzzled. 'I'll drop in again early tomorrow,' he said, 'and take some blood off you.'

Next morning he said, 'Would you think I'm mad if I said I thought you'd got subacute viral thyroiditis? I've read the chapter you wrote about de Quervain's disease in that textbook of medicine you contribute to. It seems to me you're a classic mild case. I want to see if your thyroxine level is up and whether your ESR, is raised.' (The ESR, or erythrocyte sedimentation rate, is a non-specific test which, if raised, usually indicates that you have some type of infection.)

He was right but, as you will see in a minute, there was more to come.

So if you get subacute viral thyroiditis, the illness usually starts with a generalized 'flu-like illness with tiredness, muscular aches and pains, a mild headache, and a slight fever. After a few days your thyroid gland becomes slightly but uniformly enlarged, painful, and tender to the touch. Swallowing hurts and characteristically stabs of pain run up the front of your neck to the ear on one or both sides.

Because the gland is inflamed by the virus, the pre-formed thyroid hormones leach out into the bloodstream and the levels of thyroid hormones rise. This induces the symptoms of hyperthyroidism and you become mildly thyrotoxic.

I certainly could feel my heart pounding away at 92 beats per minute even when I was resting in bed; I was sweaty and irritable. I ate well enough but lost 4 lb (1.8 kg) in the second week and rather less in the next. My hands became shaky when holding a teacup. It took me about a month to get over it, and all I took was some aspirin.

You may go to your doctor complaining of a sore throat. Unless you make it clear you mean the soreness is in the front of your neck, your doctor may mistakenly focus his attention on the pharynx at the back of your mouth and find that the tonsillar area is normal or slightly pinker than normal. Unless he perceives that it is your thyroid gland in your neck that is sore, the diagnosis may well be missed.

Most people with subacute viral thyroiditis get well in 3–6 weeks, and a stoical patient may ignore the symptoms altogether. If you have a bad attack you will be ill for rather longer, with symptoms that wax and wane, and you may feel quite ill for a time.

How is the diagnosis confirmed?

Provided the diagnosis is suspected from your history and what your doctor finds, it can easily be confirmed. During the acute inflammatory phase the blood levels of T_4 and T_3 are raised and because of the feedback mechanism your

TSH is suppressed. Usually the ESR is raised quite considerably. The sure way of distinguishing this from other causes of thyroid overactivity is to do a radio-isotope scan. Because the thyroid cells are so deranged by the inflammation caused by the virus, they do not take up much isotope. With reference to the analogy of the car factory in Chapter 3 (p. 23), this is a situation when no raw steel is going into the factory, yet more than the normal number of finished cars are coming out at the other end.

Sometimes it is necessary for your doctor to distinguish subacute viral thyroiditis from the early stages of Hashimoto's thyroiditis or from Graves' disease. In Hashimoto's disease there is a high level of thyroid autoantibodies. In Graves' disease the gland is rarely tender and the uptake of radio-isotope is increased, not reduced as in viral thyroiditis.

Treatment

If you have mild de Quervain's disease you may need no treatment beyond aspirin, paracetamol (acetaminophen), or a non-steroidal anti-inflammatory drug, such as ibuprofen, to relieve the discomfort in your neck. If the symptoms of thyrotoxicosis are troublesome, treatment with a beta-blocker is usually adequate to control them. If the discomfort in your neck is not controlled by simple analgesics, prednisone or prednisolone (cortisone-like drugs) reduces the inflammation in your thyroid gland. Initially you will probably be given a fairly large dose (30–40 mg daily) for the first week and then the amount is gradually reduced over the next 3–6 weeks. Some people experience a relapse and the course of steroids has to be repeated.

It is unusual for the thyroid gland to be damaged permanently, although after the acute phase you may have temporary thyroid deficiency for a time.

Questions and Answers

Q.1　The two lots of tablets you gave me last week have helped, doctor. I'm in much less of a state and my heart is not banging around, but my neck still hurts a lot. In fact I think it's more painful than it was and swallowing hurts. Is there anything you can do?

A. The beta-blocker, the propranolol, I gave you is obviously helping. That's why your heart is quieter and you're not so het up. But I'am afraid the paracetamol (acetaminophen) is not strong enough to relieve your pain. I'll have to give you some prednisone for a month or 6 weeks.

Q.2 Is this form of thyroiditis going to cause permanent damage?

A. Almost certainly not. Most people get over subacute viral thyroiditis without permanent damage. There is a very faint chance that your thyroid gland might become underactive, but in that case we can easily correct the deficiency.

Q.3 Can you tell me why I've got this disease?

A. Not really. It's caused by a virus, but I don't know which virus and there's no point in trying to find out because even if I knew there's no treatment that is effective against the viruses that cause subacute viral thyroiditis.

Q.4 My husband or the children won't catch this disease from me, will they?

A. I've never heard of one member of the family catching it from another, but I know of a family in which one of the children got mumps and a month later the mother got the same condition as you have.

10
Simple non-toxic goitre

'Simple non-toxic goitre' is a time-honoured clinical description of a particular type of goitre. However, the term is not ideal. It does not indicate the cause of the condition nor, on its face value, is 'simple' appropriate.

Simple

The word 'simple' is something of a misnomer because there is nothing 'simple' about a simple non-toxic goitre! In this context the word 'simple' implies several things: that the gland is not nodular but diffusely and uniformly enlarged; that it is not hard; that it is not cancerous; and that seldom are there complications.

Non-toxic

This means that a patient with a simple non-toxic goitre has no evidence, either clinically or on laboratory testing, of hyperthyroidism. This distinguishes a simple non-toxic goitre from a goitre caused by Graves' disease (Chapter 4). Nor is there underactivity of the thyroid gland due to the 'toxicity' of an autoimmune process such as occurs in Hashimoto's thyroiditis (Chapter 7).

Goitre

'Goitre' simply means enlargement of your thyroid gland. This is easy enough to establish if you discover that your thyroid is enlarged when you are fixing the collar of your blouse or shirt in the mirror, or your friends or relatives notice it.

The size of the normal thyroid gland varies in different parts of the world, being larger in areas where there is iodine deficiency. In the Western world in a young woman with a long, thin neck the thyroid may just be visible if she holds her chin up but in most people the gland is invisible. An obvious goitre will be visible and the gland feels larger than normal. The most accurate way of defining the size of a goitre is by an ultrasound scan (sonogram). The two lobes of a thyroid gland may vary in their dimensions but, using ultrasound, a normal gland can be shown to have a total volume no greater than about 20 cubic centimetres.

Some enlargement of the thyroid gland, whether due to a simple non-toxic goitre or other causes, is quite common. In a survey done in the north-east of England a few years ago nearly 15 per cent of the population had a small or obvious goitre, with a female to male ratio of 4 to 1, which emphasizes how much more common thyroid enlargement is in women.

Do not be alarmed if you develop a goitre and do not think that you have got cancer. Thyroid cancer is a very rare disease and is by far the least common cause of generalized enlargement of the thyroid.

What do you feel?

Many people with a small, non-toxic goitre are unaware of its presence and have no symptoms. Understandably you may become apprehensive if you see in the mirror that your thyroid gland is enlarged, or a relative points this out. A few people immediately complain of 'a lump in the throat', difficulty in swallowing or a choking feeling. Because quite large goitres seldom cause any symptoms at all, it is usual that any symptoms in those with a small goitre are more the consequences of apprehension than related to the actual enlargement of the thyroid gland. Thus the investigation of someone with a simple non-toxic goitre is as important in allaying their fears as it is in determining the cause of the thyroid enlargement and deciding how best to treat it.

In the Western world the condition is most common in women aged 15–25. Over the years the gland may fluctuate in size a little but with the passage of time it tends to grow larger.

What your doctor finds

Initially a simple non-toxic goitre is seldom large, although it may be obvious. It is symmetrical, and feels smooth and soft. It is painless. Often it gradually gets smaller and may disappear altogether in time so that it can safely be left alone. If, however, whatever is causing the goitre persists, the goitre may become larger and, as the years pass, more irregular so that eventually it contains several nodules and becomes a multinodular goitre (see Chapter 11).

Complications

Any complications from a simple non-toxic goitre are unusual unless over the years the goitre increases very much in size.

Pressure symptoms

Left untreated a simple goitre may, rarely, grow to sufficient size to cause pressure symptoms by virtue of its bulk. The large veins in the neck, bringing blood back to the heart from the head, may become compressed and engorged. The veins then stand out on one or both sides of your neck, and you may have a sense of fullness in the face with puffiness below the eyes.

The windpipe may be compressed if the goitre becomes very large and especially if part of the goitre lies behind the breast-bone (p. 1). The windpipe may be pushed to one side and compressed if your thyroid becomes asymmetrical.

In extreme cases, breathing is partially obstructed and when asleep you may make a curious crowing noise, known as stridor (p. 58).

Involvement of the nerves to the vocal cords

Very seldom indeed does pressure from a simple non-toxic goitre, even a large one, impair the function of the nerves that activate your vocal cords. If you develop weakness or hoarseness of your voice, you should see your doctor forthwith.

Hypothyroidism

Over the years a simple non-toxic goitre may fail to pro-duce sufficient thyroid hormones, either because the initial cause, for example iodine deficiency, or the goitre persists, or because the gland becomes involved, as a separate ill-ness, by Hashimoto's autoimmune thyroiditis (Chapter 7).

Hyperthyroidism

Only when a simple non-toxic goitre has progressed to a multinodular goitre will thyroid overactivity sometimes develop (p. 121).

Causes of simple non-toxic goitre

'Normal' or physiological causes

Slight enlargement of the thyroid gland is common in girls at or soon after the onset of puberty, and quite a number of normal women notice that their thyroid gland becomes slightly larger around the time of their menstrual period. Enlargement of the gland is common in pregnancy too (p. 138). At the time of the menopause slight enlargement of the thyroid may also occur. Hormonal changes are largely responsible for your thyroid becoming larger under these circumstances but it has also been suggested that a minor degree of iodine deficiency may sometimes be a factor, par-ticularly in pregnancy, because when you are pregnant, the baby growing inside you needs iodine and you lose more iodine in your urine. Hence your body stores of iodine may become somewhat reduced.

Iodine deficiency and endemic goitre

World-wide iodine deficiency is the most common cause of a simple non-toxic goitre, but it only occurs in areas where there is lack of iodine in the diet or the diet contains antithyroid or goitre-producing substances (goitrogens) that interfere with the use of the small amount of iodine available and so interfere with the synthesis of thyroid hormones. It is estimated that 500 million people, most of them living in underdeveloped countries, suffer from iodine deficiency.

Iodine is essential for the manufacture of the thyroid hormones, and if iodine is in short supply the thyroid gland may enlarge under the influence of the thyroid-stimulating hormone secreted by the pituitary in an attempt, often successful, to maintain normal levels of the thyroid hormones in the bloodstream. The iodine content of food, mainly in milk, eggs, and vegetables, largely depends upon the amount of iodine in the soil, and this in turn depends upon the fall of rain derived from sea water. Thus iodine deficiency is found in areas far removed from the sea. Such was the case in alpine countries such as Switzerland, around the Great Lakes in the United States, and even in the Pennines in England ('Derbyshire neck') until corrective measures were taken to fortify salt and bread with iodine. Iodine deficiency is still common in large, land-locked areas such as the Himalayas, parts of China, Iran, the Congo basin, the Andes, and in New Guinea, where preventive measures are still imperfect. In these parts of the world goitre is so common that it effects 20 per cent or more of the population and is therefore called endemic.

In iodine-deficient regions there is a direct relationship between the degree of iodine deficiency and the prevalence of goitre. If the deficiency is marked, and this can be assessed by finding very small amounts of iodine in a

24-hour urine collection, a large proportion of the population will have a goitre. In such areas the incidence of goitre and the risk of an iodine-deficient goitrous mother giving birth to a baby with thyroid deficiency has been reduced by fortifying cooking salt with iodine and also by giving her an injection of iodized poppy-seed oil every 5 years.

Foods and drugs

Certain foods and drugs interfere with the synthesis of thyroid hormones. Cabbage, certain vegetables of the kale family, and cassava (which is consumed as a staple diet in Africa), or milk from cows that have been fed on kale, may produce a goitre. Similarly, certain medicines from your chemist, notably cough and asthma cures which may contain a large amount of iodine, cause thyroid enlargement when taken over a long period of time. Many drugs, ranging from those used for the treatment of irregularities of the heart beat, such as amiodarone, to those used to treat certain mental illnesses, such as lithium, may cause the thyroid to enlarge. If you develop a goitre, you must tell your doctor about all the drugs, medicines, or herbal remedies that you are taking or have taken during previous months.

Disturbed manufacture of thyroid hormones

The making of the thyroid hormones, thyroxine (T_4) and triiodothyronine (T_3), involves many orderly chemical steps and normally each is precisely regulated, in the same way as the assembly of a motorcar involves many distinct stages. In some people the synthesis of thyroid hormones may be slowed down at one particular stage. This is called dyshormonogenesis, a word that means literally 'disordered genesis (formation) of hormones'. The severity of the disorder may vary from a mild hiccup in the synthetic process to a more major hold-up.

Goitres caused by dyshormonogenesis are very rare and tend to run in families. Usually the condition declares itself soon after birth because the baby has a goitre. In others the abnormality does not become noticeable until some years later because as the child grows and the need for thyroid hormone increases the gland enlarges in an attempt to meet the demand. In rare instances disordered thyroid hormone synthesis is associated with other congenital problems, such as deafness, a condition known as Pendred's syndrome after the doctor who originally recognized the association.

In most of these patients treatment with thyroxine prevents the goitre from getting any larger and often makes it smaller. Furthermore, such treatment obviates the risk of the patient becoming thyroid hormone deficient.

Diagnosis of simple non-toxic goitre

Although a careful history will be taken and extensive tests may be done, it is often impossible to discover the precise cause of a simple non-toxic goitre. Thyroid function tests (the blood levels of T_4, T_3, and TSH) are normal. There is nothing from a dietary history to suggest iodine deficiency, no evidence of autoimmune thyroid disease. (i.e. no thyroid autoantibodies), and no good evidence of abnormal thyroid hormone synthesis, although this is difficult to be sure of unless you have access to a specialized research laboratory. As you will now understand, the diagnosis of simple non-toxic goitre is based on proving a lot of negatives, although when the condition runs in families, this suggests a mild form of dyshormonogenesis. Nor usually is there any history of eating peculiar foods or taking drugs that may induce a goitre. In the early stages an isotope scan will show a normal pattern of uptake.

Treatment

The logical treatment of a simple non-toxic goitre is to correct or remove the cause, but as this is unknown in most patients, it is not always possible. Most small goitres can be left alone because they are benign and likely to get smaller.

An adequate intake of iodine may be all that is required. It is sensible for you to always use iodized salt or sea-salt, both of which are widely available in supermarkets and clearly labelled as 'iodized'. These types of salt should be used in cooking and at the table. Sea-fish is also a good source of iodine. You should remain under regular observation, initially every 4 months and later every year for a few years. On the other hand, excessive amounts of iodine may cause a goitre and you should avoid taking large amounts of Kelp, seaweed, and iodine-containing medicaments.

If your gland increases in size with an adequate iodine intake—and this means neither too little or too much—or your gland is already large when you first seek medical advice, treatment with thyroxine is often used. The initial dose is usually 0.05 mg daily but this may be increased to 0.1 mg or 0.15 mg daily. This treatment is usually continued for about 6 months to see if it is effective. In some people the position remains static, but in others the thyroid shrinks.

In those who do not seek advice until the thyroid is so large that it is cosmetically unsightly or it has become a multi-nodular goitre, radio-iodine treatment or surgery may have to be considered. Both are likely to be effective if your sizeable goitre is causing compression symptoms or if the gland lies behind the breast-bone. After either treatment it will be necessary for you to take thyroxine for the rest of your life.

Questions and Answers

Q.1 What do you mean exactly when you say I've got a goitre?

A. The word goitre simply means enlargement of your thyroid gland.

Q.2 Does it mean that I've got cancer?

A. Certainly not. Most goitres are *not* malignant.

Q.3 Why have I got a goitre?

A. I don't know—yet. That is what I am going to try to find out. There are many different causes.

Q.4 Will it get any bigger? It's ugly enough as it is!

A. It's not that big and most people wouldn't notice anything wrong with you. There's a good chance that we can prevent it getting any bigger and probably it will get smaller.

11
Multinodular goitre and the solitary nodule

If you have a multinodular goitre, it is highly likely that you have had a problem with your thyroid gland for many years. On the other hand, a solitary nodule or lump in your thyroid may appear suddenly 'out of the blue'. You may have noticed a very small swelling, a lump, in your neck and ignored it, but when this suddenly increases in size and becomes really quite painful, you may seek medical advice in something of a panic.

Multinodular goitre

First let us look at a multinodular goitre. Several lumps (nodules) develop in your thyroid gland and this often happens after your thyroid has been enlarged for some years. The condition is more common in women than men. The enlargement may have evolved from a simple non-toxic goitre (Chapter 10) or be associated with Hashimoto's thyroiditis (Chapter 7). A multinodular goitre is usually the result of some low-grade, probably intermittent, stimulus to the thyroid gland, as may result from iodine deficiency, goitrogens in the diet, dyshormonogenesis (p. 116), or an autoimmune disease, which causes small groups of thyroid cells to multiply and increase in size. Multinodular goitre is quite common and in the Western world is found in about 5 per cent of women, particularly in those aged 45 or over. It is even more common in those parts of the world where there is iodine deficiency.

To be felt by you or your doctor, a nodule has to be 1 cm in diameter. Often, however, additional nodules are present which are too small to be felt, and are only revealed when an ultrasound scan of the thyroid, which can detect nodules only a few millimetres in diameter, is done. The great majority of multinodular goitres are not malignant but it may be difficult to exclude cancer with certainty unless a fine-needle aspiration is done, although this is seldom necessary.

What you feel

The enlargement of your thyroid is usually obvious. The swelling is irregular and knobbly and you may be able to feel one or more painless nodules. Some patients, particularly older women, ignore the condition and fail to seek help until the goitre is really large and is causing pressure symptoms. The most common problem then is compression of the windpipe. This may cause obvious shortness of breath or stridor (p. 58). The compression may also impede the expectoration of sputum from the lungs and bronchial tubes. The patient is then likely to have a chronic cough and is prone to bronchitis or pneumonia. With inability to 'clear' the lungs, what in an ordinary person would be a minor pulmonary infection may prove lethal. Other pressure symptoms are difficulty in swallowing, hoarseness or weakness of the voice due to pressure on the nerves to the vocal cords, and engorgement of the veins in the neck with a feeling of congestion in the face.

The magnitude of the problem is best defined by an ultrasound scan and in some patients by a CT scan which will show clearly whether the goitre is also substernal, extending downwards behind the breast-bone, or is intrathoracic (p. 1). A radio-isotope scan, done with technetium or radio-iodine, will show gross irregularity of uptake. Sometimes most of the uptake is concentrated in a few of the nodules, which are therefore described as 'hot', and the rest of the gland is 'resting' or suppressed, taking up little of the isotope. Usually the blood levels of free T_4 and T_3 and of TSH are normal, but if the nodules are 'hot' and secrete increased amounts of the thyroid hormones, the patient will be thyrotoxic.

In older patients thyrotoxicosis due to 'hot' nodules in a multinodular goitre is common and of insidious onset. The condition is sometimes called Plummer's disease after the American surgeon who distinguished it from Graves' disease. Many of these patients fail to exhibit the classic symptoms and signs seen in a younger thyrotoxic patient. They may not lose a lot of weight. They may not be particularly anxious and may not have a tremor. What they do develop is insidious congestive heart failure with an irregular pulse due to atrial fibrillation, swelling of the feet and ankles, and shortness of breath so that at night they cannot lie flat and have to sleep propped up with pillows.

Treatment

Once any question of cancer and of hyperthyroidism have been excluded, there may be no need for any special treatment if the multinodular goitre is small, although you must remain under medical surveillance. Although thyroxine was sometimes prescribed in the past, there is little evidence that this will make the multinodular goitre smaller or prevent it from becoming larger. In most instances radioiodine is the treatment of choice. A relatively large dose has to be given. This will reduce the size of a multinodular goitre by about 50 per cent after 1 year so that the appearance is cosmetically more acceptable, but of course the gland will not be of normal dimensions. Radioactive treatment will also cure any hyperthyroidism but the overactivity of the gland may first have to be controlled with an antithyroid drug.

Alternatively the goitre can be removed surgically. This is not difficult in the younger patient but is a more formidable undertaking in an elderly patient, although clearly indicated if malignant change is suggested by involvement of the laryngeal nerves to the vocal cords or the development of enlarged lymph glands in the neck.

A solitary nodule

You may develop a single nodule, which is unattached to the overlying skin and not associated with any enlargement of the lymph glands in your neck. What appears to be a single nodule may on ultrasound scanning prove to be one of several nodules which are too small to be palpable. Hence what appears to be a solitary nodule is often the first visible expression of a multinodular goitre (see above).

A solitary nodule usually appears as a smooth, rounded lump that is not painful. It may contain fluid and therefore is a cyst but this can only be established with certainty from an ultrasound scan or by doing a fine-needle aspiration when fluid will be withdrawn. Very few cysts are malignant.

Sudden painful enlargement of a nodule will occur if bleeding takes place into it. The reason for this happening is not known. The smooth round swelling increases quite suddenly in size, becomes hard because of the increased pressure inside it, and may be very painful, particularly if you press on it. If a fine-needle aspiration is done (p. 33), blood-stained fluid will be withdrawn; the lump then becomes less tense and the pain is relieved.

A single nodule is usually a benign, non-toxic cluster of cells—benign because it is not cancerous and non-toxic because it does not produce an excess of thyroid hormones. However, a benign non-toxic nodule may over the years begin to produce excess thyroid hormones and you become thyrotoxic. This is discussed above and in Chapter 6.

Unless it causes obvious symptoms of thyrotoxicosis, confirmed by thyroid function tests, a nodule must always be shown not to be malignant. The distinction between benign and cancerous is not easy and three procedures, some more reliable than others, are used to decide this:

1. A fine-needle aspiration (p. 33) is the best. Seldom does it fail to produce enough cells for accurate assessment. Occasionally the appearance of the cells under the microscope may be questionable and not allow total exclusion of cancer. If this happens, another fine-needle aspiration biopsy must be done.

2. An ultrasound scan (p. 34) will show whether the nodule is filled with fluid and is therefore cystic, which makes it more likely to be benign. Otherwise, ultrasound scans are unreliable in distinguishing between benign or malignant nodules.

3. An isotope scan with either radio-iodine or technetium may show some uptake in a benign nodule but usually little or no uptake in a cancerous one. Certainly a 'cold' nodule, which does not take up the isotope, is more suspicious of cancer than a 'warm' or 'hot' one, but many benign lumps and cysts are 'cold' and only about 10 per cent of 'cold' nodules turn out to be cancerous. If the isotope scan shows that in fact you have several nodules, this makes it even more unlikely that you have cancer. It must be emphasized that nodules are much more often benign than cancerous.

Because these tests for distinguishing between a benign isolated nodule and a cancerous one are not always conclusive, do not be upset if your doctor advises surgical removal of the lump or of the lobe containing the lump (a hemithyroidectomy). Not only will this establish the precise diagnosis with certainty but the surgery will hopefully get rid of your problem permanently.

Questions and Answers

Q.1   Is this little lump that has developed in my neck likely to be cancer?

A.   The lump is in your thyroid gland and is not an enlarged lymph gland. It's unlikely to be malignant but I cannot be sure until certain tests have been done.

Q.2   Are the tests you're going to do always conclusive?

A.   Not always. If not, I may have to advise you to have an operation. However, I can tell you that rather less than a quarter of patients like you have to undergo surgery.

Q.3   This lump in my neck has suddenly blown up and it really hurts. What is it?

A.   You have a nodule in your thyroid gland and bleeding into it has occurred. That's why it's suddenly enlarged and become painful. If we remove the fluid from the nodule, it will relieve your pain and the nodule will become smaller and less tense. Later I'll have to do a number of tests to find out why you've developed a nodule, and if you have also got other smaller ones that cannot be felt.

Q.4   My lump has almost disappeared since you removed the fluid from it. You say it was a thyroid cyst. Will it come back again?

A.   It may; I can't promise it won't. If it does come back, there's a good chance that removing the fluid again will fix it or we could consider injecting an agent that will cause the cyst to collapse and become fibrotic.

Q.5   I have had this goitre for years and years. Why are you so concerned about it?

A.   Because you are aged 70, and goitre is pressing on your windpipe, your trachea. You've just told me that you have difficulty in breathing and keep on having chest infections. Radio-iodine treatment given under close supervision should put you right.

12 Cancer of the thyroid gland

Compared with the incidence of malignant disease else-where in the body, thyroid cancer is responsible for less than 0.5 per cent of all deaths from cancer. Thus cancer of the thyroid gland is rare. Only 5–6 people per million of the population die of this disease each year in England and Wales or in the United States. Although it may occur at any age, it is most common between the ages of 30 and 60 and, as with other thyroid disorders, it is more common in women than men.

What is the cause of thyroid cancer?

Although the precise genetic causes of thyroid cancer are unknown, previous X-ray treatment to the head, neck, or chest is a definite predisposing factor. There was a vogue before the Second World War and in the 1950s, particu-larly in certain centres in the United States, to reduce the size of enlarged tonsils and adenoids in children by X-ray therapy in preference to surgical removal. Acne of the face in adolescents was sometimes treated similarly. A signifi-cant number of children treated in this way have developed thyroid cancer 10–60 years later, and X-ray therapy for such benign conditions in childhood has long since been abandoned. Similarly the treatment by X-rays of an enlarged thymus gland or red birth-marks on the face or neck of infants may later give rise to cancer of the thyroid. Japanese survivors of the atomic bombs in 1945 have, since the late 1950s, shown an increase in malignant thyroid nodules. The explosion at an atomic power-station in Russia has led to an increased incidence of thyroid cancer, particularly in children, in the region around Chernobyl.

The liability to develop thyroid cancer after exposure to radio-iodine is very much dose-related. You need not worry if you are or ever have been given such isotopes, as ^{131}I, for diagnostic or for therapeutic purposes. There is no evidence, after the most careful scrutiny, that they increase the incidence of subsequent thyroid cancer. Nor does a pre-existing goitre, irrespective of its cause, seem to increase the risk of malignant change, because most thyroid cancers develop in a previously normal gland.

Points that may alert your doctor to the possibility of thyroid cancer are:

- a previous history of X-ray therapy to the head or neck;
- the sudden development of a lump, which may or may not be painful, in your thyroid gland;
- a lump in, or asymmetrical enlargement of, the thyroid, particularly in a child or a man (because thyroid disease is relatively uncommon in men);
- hoarseness of your voice;
- the finding of enlarged lymph glands in the neck in association with a goitre or a thyroid nodule;
- excessive hardness of the thyroid or the nodule;
- fixation of the nodule or the thyroid gland to the skin or the muscles in the neck so that it does not move freely when you swallow.

Are there different types of thyroid cancer?

There are several different types of cancers that effect the thyroid gland and these can be separated into two main groups:

- those in which the cells are well differentiated and look

and behave in rather the same way as normal thyroid cells; and

- those in which the cells are not differentiated (ana-plastic) and behave in an unruly aggressive manner.

Differentiated cancers

There are two distinctive types of differentiated thyroid cancers. The most common is the papillary type which tends to affect children and young women, and spreads to the neighbouring lymph glands in the neck. It is liable to occur in several sites in the thyroid gland at the same time. The other type is the follicular cell cancer which mainly occurs in women over 30 and tends to spread to the lungs or bones.

In both types the cells that have become malignant continue to look very much like normal thyroid cells and behave like them too. They continue to respond to the thyroid-stimulating hormone from the pituitary and they usually continue to take up iodine (and radio-iodine) from the bloodstream. Therefore these tumours are relatively 'civilized'; they grow slowly and spread to distant parts of the body (metastasize) late. The fact that they continue to take up radio-iodine makes the detection of secondary deposits (metastases) in other parts of the body easier and allows effective treatment to be given by irradiating the metastases with radio-iodine. Also, if the secretion of TSH from the pituitary is reduced to negligible amounts by giving sufficient thyroxine by mouth, the stimulus for any residual cancer cells to grow is diminished.

Undifferentiated cancers

Less commonly the cells of a thyroid cancer are un-differentiated. These 'uncivilized' anaplastic cells, like anarchists, are uncontrolled and uncontrollable. They multiple rapidly and invade surrounding structures in the neck, which may make surgical removal difficult or impossible.

There are certain other forms of cancer that may involve the thyroid gland and these are mentioned for the sake of completeness.

Medullary cell cancer

A very rare form of cancer may develop from cells which, strictly speaking, are not thyroid cells at all but 'lodgers' living in the thyroid gland. These so-called medullary cells, also known as C cells or parafollicular cells, do not make or secrete thyroid hormones. They manufacture a hormone called calcitonin (hence 'C cells') which regulates the amount of calcium in your bones. They may also secrete other hormones that increase the activity of the intestines and cause diarrhoea. These rare medullary cell cancers tend to run in families and may be associated with small, non-malignant tumours of the adrenal glands in the abdomen (phaeochromocytomas) that secrete excess adrenaline (epinephrine) and noradrenaline (norepinephrine)—hormones that cause high blood pressure. Because so rare, medullary-cell cancers will not be considered further except to say that surgical removal of first the associated benign phaeochromocytoma(s) in the abdomen and then the malignant tumour in the neck is usually effective and successful.

Lymphomas

Sometimes the thyroid is the site of a malignant lymphoma, a tumour that arises from white corpuscles (lymphocytes or related cells) residing in the thyroid gland. Lymphomas are often fast growing so that the thyroid increases rapidly in size and may compress the windpipe to cause shortness of breath or a crowing noise (stridor) when you breathe. These tumours are usually sensitive to X-ray treatment and chemotherapy.

Metastatic cancer

Sometimes the thyroid becomes the site of a single or multiple secondary deposits from a primary cancer in the lung, breast, or kidney, but at this stage the underlying growth will usually have declared itself.

What happens to you in thyroid cancer?

If you develop one of the most common differentiated types of thyroid cancer—the papillary or follicular varieties— the first thing you will probably notice is a small lump in your thyroid gland. This lump is usually round and nodular, often hard to the touch, usually but not always painless, and may initially be little bigger than a small grape. If you have a papillary thyroid cancer, more than one nodule may appear simultaneously. The malignant cells may spread to a nearby lymph gland in your neck. This enlarged lymph gland may be what first takes you to your doctor, who finds a painless enlarged lymph node with little to suggest, until he makes a careful examination, that you have a primary growth in your thyroid.

Left untreated a papillary differentiated thyroid cancer will eventually spread (metastasize) to other parts of your body, the malignant cells being carried in the bloodstream or the lymphatic system to your lungs, liver, or your bones. Not until there has been considerable destruction of a bone by a metastasis will you feel any bone pain. Sometimes the pain comes on suddenly if the involved bone breaks without a preceding fall or unusual force being applied (a 'pathological fracture'). Hoarseness of your voice may also occur if the malignant cells encroach on the nerves that activate your vocal cords.

The undifferentiated anaplastic type of thyroid cancer tends to occur in older people. The thyroid gland enlarges quite quickly and becomes generally tender. The highly malignant cells may invade the overlying skin, making it red as though it were inflamed. Deeper structures in your neck may be invaded so that on swallowing your thyroid gland does not move up and down in your neck as freely as it should. Huskiness of the voice is common.

How is cancer of the thyroid diagnosed?

The diagnosis is made on the basis of your doctor's clinical suspicion and confirmed by a fine-needle aspiration. If this is inconclusive, the diagnosis may be confirmed only by surgery. Sometimes additional tests are done but they are usually less informative.

A radio-iodine scan is of limited help in deciding that cancer is probably *not* present but is less helpful in deciding that it is. Malignant tissue often fails to take up the isotope as avidly as do normal thyroid cells and are therefore 'cold'. Although many benign lumps do take up the isotope, unfortunately many do not and are also 'cold'. Thus if your lump takes up the isotope, it is less likely to be a cancer. If it fails to do so, however, it could be either malignant or benign. If the isotope scan shows numerous nodules, you probably have a benign multinodular goitre and not a cancer (p. 121). An ultrasound scan is seldom very helpful, although a cyst is less likely to be malignant than a solid lesion. Tests of thyroid function may be done but these are usually normal and of little help in establishing the diagnosis. Only rarely is a thyroid cancer, even when it has spread widely, the cause of thyrotoxicosis or thyroid failure.

An enlarged lymph node in the neck

There are many relatively trivial and also some serious causes for you developing an enlarged lymph node in the neck. Happily the less serious causes are much more common than the serious ones. They range from a simple sore throat or glandular fever (infective mononucleosis) to tuberculosis, other infective diseases, and cancer of various kinds. Examination by your doctor and simple investigations will usually establish the cause but sometimes more complicated tests are required, including the removal of the lymph gland for microscopic examination.

How is cancer of the thyroid treated?

Differentiated cancer

The treatment of a differentiated thyroid cancer is usually successful. At operation, while you are anaesthetized, the tissue under suspicion is removed and examined under a microscope. This will usually allow a distinction between a papillary or follicular carcinoma, but this is not always easy for the pathologist.

If you have a follicular cancer, the surgeon will probably remove only the lobe of the thyroid containing it (a hemithyroidectomy). If you have the more common papillary cancer, the surgeon will remove all your thyroid gland or as much of it as he safely can. This is done because of the possibility that additional small areas of cancer may be present in other parts of the thyroid gland. In skilled hands a total or near-total thyroidectomy can usually be accomplished without damage to the nerves to your vocal cords and without loss of your parathyroid glands (p. 57). The surgeon will remove any neighbouring lymph glands in your neck, which may be the site of local spread.

Some few weeks after you have recovered from the operation, whether you have had a papillary or follicular type of cancer, but particularly with a papillary one, you will be given a large therapeutic dose of radioactive iodine with the objective of killing off any residual thyroid cells—normal or malignant. This will mean being admitted to hospital where you will be nursed in a special room. After you have been given the therapeutic dose of radio-iodine, the radioactivity in your body will be carefully monitored and you will be discharged from hospital after about a week when the radiation has fallen to an acceptable level. You will be advised when you can resume non-essential contact with children and other adults, and when you can return to work.

Thereafter you will be given thyroxine, not only as replacement therapy for your inevitable thyroid deficiency but also to suppress the level of TSH in your bloodstream and so reduce the stimulus for any remaining cancer cells to grow. The dosage of thyroxine will be adjusted until the level of your TSH is below normal, but the dosage will not be sufficient to make you hyperthyroid. By keeping the TSH level suppressed any remaining malignant thyroid cells are not exposed to its stimulating action; thus they remain dormant.

After 6–9 months your hospital doctor will check that all is well with you. Nowadays, at regular intervals of 6–12 months, he will monitor your freedom from any recurrence of the cancer by measuring the level of thyroglobulin in your blood. This is a substance normally present in small amounts in healthy people and is manufactured by normal and malignant thyroid cells. In patients with a differentiated thyroid cancer, either papillary or follicular, which has been treated in the way described above, a negligible amount of thyroglobulin should be found in your blood because all the normal and malignant thyroid cells have been eradicated. Increased amounts of thyroglobulin will appear if there is a recurrence of your cancer. Thus your doctor will simply monitor your thyroglobulin level while you continue taking thyroxine to prevent thyroid deficiency and to suppress your TSH.

If the thyroglobulin level rises, your replacement thyroid hormone treatment will be stopped for a few weeks until your TSH level has risen above the upper normal range. Then you will be given a dose of radio-iodine and a scan done of your neck and whole body. If any significant number of thyroid cells, normal or malignant, remain in the neck they will show up and so also will any significant number of differentiated cancerous cells that have formed secondary deposits elsewhere in your body.

If the scans show evidence of residual thyroid tissue, another therapeutic dose of radio-iodine is given and the replacement treatment with thyroid hormone resumed.

Before measurement of the blood thyroglobulin level was introduced, a radio-iodine scan was, and in some centres still is, repeated annually so that any recurrence of the cancer could be detected early and treated with a therapeutic dose of [131]I.

Undifferentiated thyroid cancer

This type of tumour occurs predominantly in patients aged 50 or more. In the early stages of an undifferentiated (anaplastic) thyroid cancer it may be possible to remove the growth surgically, but often the best treatment is deep X-ray therapy.

Here is an account by a woman patient who had a differentiated thyroid cancer. Initially this was not treated in an ideal way but happily all is well now.

When I was aged 35 a small painless lump appeared in my thyroid gland but I took no notice of it. Two years later I had my last (my third) child and during this pregnancy the lump increased in size. Not until I was 40 did the lump seem sufficiently large for me to draw my doctor's attention to it. At that time we were living abroad. The lump was removed surgically and I was told it was a cancer. I was given thyroxine tablets.

Four years later—we were still living in Africa—I noticed another lump in my thyroid gland on the other side. This time the surgeon removed all my thyroid gland and I was given more thyroid hormone to take by mouth.

When I was 46 we came back to England and I noticed a painless lump in the right side of my neck under the angle of my jaw. A radio-iodine scan showed it was thyroid tissue—almost certainly malignant they said—in a lymph gland. I was operated on and several lymph glands containing cancer were removed. I was then given what my doctor said was a curative dose of radio-active iodine.

I am now 56. Isotope scans were done each year until I was 50 but now my thyroglobulin is measured every 6 months. I have had no recurrence and certainly I feel fine taking 0.25 mg thyroxine daily.

Questions and Answers

Q.1   I have had many tests and have been told that the results are encouraging, but I've been advised to have an operation. I don't understand why.

A.   The tests may indicate that your thyroid is functioning normally but the biopsy may still be equivocal and it may not be absolutely certain that this lump in your thyroid gland is not malignant. The only way to be sure is to remove it. Even if it is a cancer, the outlook is very good.

Q.2   Will I have to go through all this again next year—I mean this radio-isotope scan—to show I've not got any cancer left?

A.   No, in future your freedom from disease can be monitored by measuring a substance called thyroglobulin in a simple blood sample. Only if this test comes back positive will you have to have another radio-iodine scan.

Q.3   My dose of thyroxine has been increased. Does that mean I'm worse; that the cancer has come back?

A.   Certainly not. Your dosage of thyroxine has been raised a little because the blood level of TSH, that stimulates any remaining thyroid cells, is not sufficiently suppressed.

Q.4   But won't increasing my thyroxine dose make me nervous and jumpy?

A.   The aim is to increase the blood level of your thyroid hormone to the upper limit of normal, but not to a level that will upset you.

Q.5   Is it certain that I haven't got cancer?

A.   The ultrasound scan shows that you have a great many nodules in your thyroid, although you can feel only one. This makes it less likely to be malignant but a fine-needle aspiration of the big nodule and of other areas will be done to clarify the situation.

13
Thyroid problems during and after pregnancy

Changes in your thyroid gland and in thyroid hormone secretion occur during pregnancy, in parallel with the other major hormone adjustments that occur at this time. If you have a normal thyroid gland, these changes are of no clinical importance to you personally although your doctor, and particularly your obstetrician, will be aware that the levels of your thyroid hormones and of the thyroid stimulating hormone change during pregnancy.

Thyroid changes that occur in pregnancy

As soon as conception occurs a hormone is secreted from the placenta. This is called human chorionic gonadotrophin (hCG) because it is secreted by cells in the chorion or placenta and it stimulates the secretion of hormones, such as oestrogens, from the gonad (ovary). The oestrogens increase the blood level of thyroxine-binding thyroglobulin (TBG) by increasing the synthesis of this protein in your liver. TBG is an important protein to which thyroxine (T_4) and triiodothyronine (T_3) are bound and carried around in the bloodstream (see p. 6). In pregnancy the amount of TBG nearly doubles: more thyroxine has to be secreted by the thyroid gland to occupy the binding sites on this transport protein, otherwise the level of *free* T_4 in your bloodstream, which is the hormone that is metabolically active, might become too low.

Thus in pregnancy the thyroid gland has to produce more thyroid hormones, and there is a tendency for the gland to enlarge. The degree of this enlargement tends to vary according to the amount of iodine, which is an essential constituent of the thyroxine molecule, that is available in your body. Iodine is also necessary to supply the growing baby with this essential element, and during pregnancy you lose more iodine in your urine than normally. In countries such as the United States and most parts of the United Kingdom, where there is sufficient iodine in the diet, little or no enlargement of the thyroid gland occurs. In many parts of the world where the amount of dietary iodine is marginally or very deficient, the thyroid gland enlarges and the extent of this is related to the degree of iodine insufficiency. For example, in ancient Egypt, where dietary iodine was insufficient, a fine thread used to be tied round the neck of a young bride: when the thread broke it was taken as evidence that she had become pregnant.

Another factor that tends to make the thyroid gland larger during pregnancy is that the human chorionic gonadotrophin hormone (hCG) stimulates the thyroid gland in much the same way as the thyroid-stimulating hormone (TSH) normally does. This may increase the level of thyroid hormones in the blood, and cause some temporary lowering of the TSH level during the first 3 months but seldom below the normal range for the non-pregnant woman. Occasionally when the blood level of hCG is very high for a prolonged period of time, a pregnant woman may develop temporary hyperthyroidism (see below).

Any slight enlargement of your thyroid gland during pregnancy is unlikely to be of any consequence but you must ensure that you have an adequate—neither too little or too much—intake of iodine by using sea-salt or iodized salt in cooking and at the table, and eating sea-fish at least once a week.

Thyroid function tests during normal pregnancy

The results of thyroid function tests change during pregnancy. Because of the marked rise in the thyroxine-binding globulin, the levels of total T_4 and total T_3 rise. However, the unbound free T_4 and free T_3, which are the biologically active hormones, do not increase. Indeed, particularly during the first 3 months of pregnancy, the level of free T_4 is significantly lower than in non-pregnant women, and in one-third of pregnant women the free T_4 level is near or below the lower limit of the normal non-pregnant range. The TSH level, as explained above, may be transiently depressed during the first trimester of pregnancy when the hCG level reaches its peak, and in some 20 per cent of normal pregnant women the TSH value falls below the lower limit of normal at this time. Thereafter the TSH level tends to rise progressively until term and this is particularly common where iodine intake is restricted. Such changes are not relevant if your thyroid is normal, but they become important if you suffered from over- or underactivity of your thyroid gland before you became pregnant or if either condition is first diagnosed during your pregnancy.

Overactivity of the thyroid gland during pregnancy

Graves' disease

By far the most common cause of overactivity of the thyroid gland, of sufficient degree to induce symptoms during pregnancy, is Graves' disease. If you have untreated hyperthyroidism, you are less likely to become pregnant. However, once your overactive gland is controlled by an antithyroid drug or you are cured and made euthyroid by either surgery or radio-iodine, your fertility will be restored to normal.

Sometimes Graves' disease develops for the first time *during* pregnancy. The diagnosis is not always easy because some of the symptoms of thyroid overactivity—such as an increased heart rate and palpitations, feeling hot, increased perspiration, and tiredness—also occur in pregnant women with a normally functioning thyroid gland. An important clue may be that when you become pregnant you fail to gain weight to the expected degree or you may even lose weight.

Diagnosis of Graves' disease during pregnancy

The diagnosis is confirmed by the level of *free* thyroid hormones in your blood and a very suppressed level of TSH which is well below the lower limit of the normal range. In some centres the autoimmune cause of your Graves' disease, the thyroid-stimulating antibody (TSAb), is also measured (see p. 27). A radio-iodine uptake scan (see p. 27) must not be done because the isotope would also be taken up by the thyroid gland of the baby in your womb.

Treatment of Graves' disease during pregnancy

If you become pregnant while you are taking an antithyroid drug (see p. 53) for your Graves' disease, this treatment will be continued with the smallest effective dose during your pregnancy. Generally, propylthiouracil is preferred to carbimazole or methimazole for treating Graves' disease in pregnancy because less propylthiouracil crosses the placenta, so is less likely to suppress thyroid function in your baby. Almost certainly, except in very severe cases, the antithyroid drug can be stopped during the last 2 months of your pregnancy. In most cases this is possible because the autoimmune disorder that causes your Graves' disease tends to lessen during this time and the severity of the thyrotoxicosis becomes milder. Alternatively surgical removal of seven-eighths of your thyroid can be done during the fourth, fifth, or sixth month of your pregnancy, when it is safe to operate on you without harming your baby or risk inducing a miscarriage.

After delivery

You are likely to have a recurrence of your Graves' disease 3–6 months after delivery, and your antithyroid drug is likely to have to be re-started. Propylthiouracil is preferred to carbimazole or methimazole because less of it is secreted in your milk. However, the amount of antithyroid drug in your milk is usually very little and there is no absolute contraindication to you feeding your baby provided the baby has his or her free T_4 and TSH levels measured every 4–6 weeks.

Gestational hyperthyroidism

This is a transient episode of mild thyrotoxicosis that occurs early in pregnancy and is caused by an excessively high level of hCG which stimulates your thyroid gland. This is a rare condition, often not diagnosed because it is mild and occurs in only some 2 per cent of women. Seldom is any treatment necessary but, if the symptoms are troublesome, short-term administration of carbimazole is effective.

Hyperthyroidism in hyperemesis gravidarum

Many pregnant women suffer from morning sickness. Sometimes, however, vomiting becomes so severe that the patient becomes dehydrated and has to be admitted to hospital for replacement of the lost fluid. This condition is known as hyperemesis gravidarum (excess vomiting in the pregnant woman). It is probable that the vomiting is induced by the high levels of hCG secreted by the placenta and the high levels of oestrogens induced by the hCG. The hCG stimulates the thyroid gland, as explained above, and many patients with hyperemesis gravidarum have a degree of hyperthyroidism with raised levels of free T_4 and free T_3 and a suppressed TSH level. In addition to correction of the dehydration in hyperemesis gravidarum, treatment of the temporary hyperthyroidism with carbimazole may be necessary. The condition is usually self-limiting and the free

T_4 and free T_3 levels return to normal within a few weeks of cessation of the vomiting.

Pregnancy and the underactive thyroid gland

Infertility is common in women who have an underactive thyroid gland. Once the thyroid deficiency is corrected, however, normal fertility is restored. It is most important, if you have an underactive thyroid gland and are being given thyroid hormone replacement therapy, that you continue this during your pregnancy and afterwards. Just because your total T_4 and T_3 levels increase above the normal non-pregnant range, this is no reason to stop or reduce your dose of hormone replacement, because the free thyroid hormone levels will be normal. Furthermore, in a hypothyroid patient on treatment, the thyroid stimulating hormone (TSH) may rise during pregnancy. It may be necessary to increase the dose of thyroxine early in your pregnancy. This additional supplement may have to be further increased later in your pregnancy, and the correct amount can only be judged by your doctor measuring the free T_4 and TSH every 4–6 weeks.

Maternal thyroid problems after delivery

Abnormalities of thyroid function are common after delivery, and usually occur during the first 6 months after your baby is born. During this postpartum period either mild hyperthyroidism, hypothyroidism, or thyroid overactivity followed by underactivity may occur. As many as about 15 per cent of women, particularly those who have certain thyroid antibodies (microsomal or thyroid peroxidase antibodies, see p. 174) present in the blood before they become pregnant, develop some disorder of thyroid function during the first 6 months after having a baby. Short-lived thyroid overactivity alone, or transient thyroid overactivity followed by short-lived underactivity are less common than hypothyroidism alone.

The symptoms produced by these abnormalities are not always recognized because many women accept them as the consequences of having to look after a new baby and having to run their home. Often the thyroid over- or underactivity is so short lived that no treatment is necessary.

Maternal hypothyroidism after delivery

About 10 per cent of apparently normal, healthy women are found to have thyroid autoantibodies in the blood when they first attend an antenatal clinic. Although there is a slightly increased risk of you having a miscarriage if you have these antibodies, they seldom cause any problems during pregnancy. After delivery the symptoms of underactivity of the thyroid gland, characterized by fatigue, weakness, depression, failure to lose weight, impairment of memory, and lack of ability to concentrate may occur and may incorrectly be attributed to postpartum 'blues'. Treatment with thyroxine is very helpful. In some women the thyroxine replacement is only required temporarily but in about a quarter it is required on a permanent basis.

Maternal hyperthyroidism after delivery due to silent thyroiditis

Postpartum thyroiditis causing hyperthyroidism is usually so short-lived that no treatment is required, although if necessary a beta-blocker (p. 49) will help relieve any symptoms. Postpartum hyperthyroidism is also known as 'silent thyroiditis' (p. 151)—'silent' not because there are no symptoms but because the thyroid gland is not painful or tender and seldom is it obviously enlarged. This thyroid overactivity is due to a type of autoimmune thyroiditis quite distinct from Graves' disease and only partially related to Hashimoto's thyroiditis. Radio-iodine scanning shows reduced uptake of the isotope, but this test can only be done if you stop breast-feeding for 4 days because the radioactive iodine may be secreted in your milk. Silent thyroiditis is discussed further in Chapter 14.

Neonatal hyperthyroidism

Thyroid overactivity in a new-born baby (congenital hyperthyroidism) is very rare. It occurs only when the baby's mother was successfully treated for Graves' disease in the past or has had Graves' disease during her recent pregnancy. The cause of the baby's hyperthyroidism is the thyroid-stimulating antibody that you have in your blood and which is passed, during pregnancy, to your baby. These stimulating antibodies may persist in your blood even though your Grave's disease was treated and cured long ago.

In fact very few babies (less than 1 in a 100) of previous thyrotoxic mothers are affected, but they are somewhat more likely to be so if you had severe eye complications (Chapter 5) or pretibial myxoedema (p. 43)—both findings that may be associated with high levels of thyroid stimulating antibodies that may persist in your blood.

If you were treated with an antithyroid drug during pregnancy it is unlikely your baby will be born hyperthyroid because the propylthiouracil, carbimazole, or methimazole will cross the placenta and tend to suppress your baby's thyroid gland.

Predicting neonatal hyperthyroidism

In women with a past or present history of Graves' disease, a careful watch will be kept on your baby before it is born. Congenital hyperthyroidism may be suspected if *in utero* your baby's heart rate is unduly fast or if your baby grows abnormally fast as measured by ultrasound scans. Your doctor may be alerted to the possibility of your baby being thyrotoxic by finding a high level of thyroid-stimulating antibodies in your blood. Where this test is available it should be done if you have Graves' disease during your pregnancy or you had it in the past. If there is evidence of intrauterine thyrotoxicosis, the overactive thyroid of your baby can be treated by giving you an antithyroid drug which will cross the placenta. During this treatment you yourself can be prevented from becoming hypothyroid by being given thyroxine which barely crosses the placenta and thus will not affect your baby.

Congenital hyperthyroidism

If, as rarely happens, your new-born baby has congenital hyperthyroidism, he or she will have an unduly fast heart rate and be restless. Minimal eye signs may be present but the main other features are failure to thrive and gain weight despite an enormous appetite, flushing of the skin, and possibly diarrhoea. Your baby's thyroid gland is likely to be enlarged but this is not easy to detect at this age. The diagnosis can be confirmed quickly by measuring your baby's thyroid hormone levels, but it must be remembered that a mildly raised T_4 level is normal within the first week of birth.

Treatment is given with small doses of iodine or an antithyroid drug. Fortunately, neonatal thyrotoxicosis is self-limiting because the thyroid-stimulating antibodies from you persist in your baby for only a few weeks or months. Thus active treatment is only required during this time.

Neonatal hypothyroidism

If you were given an antithyroid drug during your pregnancy to control your Graves' disease, in theory your baby could be born with a suppressed thyroid gland, but this is unlikely. Under these circumstances thyroid deficiency in the newborn is rare.

If you developed hypothyroidism during your pregnancy and were treated for this, you need not worry. Do not forget that your baby has its own thyroid gland that started working when it was an 8-week-old fetus.

However, like every other baby, yours must be tested to exclude thyroid deficiency around the fifth day after birth (p. 97–8) because the more common cause of hypothyroidism, lack of thyroid tissue, could affect your baby like anyone else's, and this occurs in approximately 1 in 3500 births.

Questions and Answers

Q.1 After my first baby was born, I had thyroid deficiency for about 4 months. Is this likely to happen again if I have another child?

A. Yes, it is, particularly as we know that you have thyroid autoantibodies in your blood.

Q.2 Would it be better to have an operation for my Graves' disease when I am 4 or 5 months pregnant or go on taking an antithyroid drug all the way through my pregnancy?

A. The choice must be yours, but I think it unlikely you would need to take an antithyroid drug all through your pregnancy. We shall probably stop it 6–8 weeks before you've delivered. You are likely to have to restart it again within 3 months of delivery.

Q.3 My obstetrician asked me to tell you that my thyroxine level is too high. He wondered whether I should reduce my dose of thyroxine to the amount I was having before I became pregnant.

A. The level of your *total* thyroxine is high, but that always happens in pregnancy. I'll measure your free thyroxine and your TSH. If they're normal, you should go on with the present dose. I'll let you know the results.

Q.4. Will there be problems in feeding my baby if I am on an antithyroid drug?

A. Not really. A tiny amount of the antithyroid drug may be present in your milk. This is unlikely to affect your baby but we shall be on the lookout for this.

Q.5.   You've told me I have Graves' disease. I feel fine on treatment but will my baby be all right?

A.   You are having the smallest dose of the antithyroid drug, propylthiouracil, to control your hyperthyroidism and this can usually be stopped altogether a few weeks before your baby is born. It is unlikely to harm your baby.

14
Miscellaneous disorders of the thyroid gland

A number of miscellaneous disorders of the thyroid gland, not adequately dealt with elsewhere in this book or in need of further consideration, are discussed in this chapter.

Pituitary diseases and the thyroid

Although the relationship between the pituitary gland, its secretion of thyroid-stimulating hormone (TSH), and the thyroid gland have been discussed in Chapter 1, little mention has been made of the thyroid disorders that may develop as a consequence of pituitary disease.

Excessive secretion of TSH from the pituitary

Overactivity of the pituitary gland with increased secretion of TSH is a rare cause of thyroid overactivity (p. 80). The clue that leads to your doctor diagnosing this is that you are thyrotoxic with a raised level of thyroid hormones in your blood, but surprisingly the TSH level is normal or raised—not suppressed as is usually the case due to operation of the feedback mechanism (p. 5). When increased T_4 or T_3 production is caused by a disorder that is primarily in the thyroid gland, the raised level of thyroid hormones switches off the pituitary secretion of TSH.

Although antithyroid drugs will reduce the excessive production of thyroid hormones caused by excess TSH secretion from the pituitary and will render you euthyroid, this treatment will not cure the underlying condition. Attention has to be given to why your pituitary gland is secreting too much TSH. The cause is usually a benign pituitary tumour which is best removed surgically by an operation that is done through your nose.

Reduced secretion of TSH by the pituitary gland

Failure of the pituitary gland to secrete enough TSH is more common and is the cause of secondary, as opposed to primary, thyroid failure. Lack of enough TSH reduces the secretion of thyroid hormones from your thyroid gland, and causes a clinical picture very similar to that which follows primary failure of the thyroid gland (Chapter 8). This picture is often modified, however, by additional features resulting from the diminished secretion of other pituitary hormones that influence growth, sexual development and function, and the adrenal glands.

Reduced secretion of TSH is usually due to either a tumour or some other damage to your pituitary gland. Thus in addition to failure of your thyroid, there is failure of the other endocrine glands which are regulated by your pituitary. If a tumour of the pituitary is the cause, it may induce local symptoms, such as headaches and/or visual disturbances because the nerves that carry the signals from your eyes to the brain pass close to the pituitary gland.

If a tumour is present, treatment must be directed at this and replacement therapy also given, not only to make good the thyroid deficiency but the deficiencies of the other endocrine glands that are controlled by the pituitary, such as the ovaries in women, the testes in men, and the adrenal glands—all of which are likely to be underactive too.

Here is an account of the illness of a woman who suffered destruction of her pituitary gland as a result of an unhappy obstetric event. In pregnancy the pituitary gland enlarges and is very dependent on a good blood supply. As we shall learn this patient's blood supply to her pituitary was jeopardized when she had her baby.

I'm now 39 years old. I got married at the age of 26 after training to be a nurse. My husband is a lawyer and we moved to the Middle East where I had Benjamin when I was 28. Immediately after he was born I had an enormous haemorrhage. The head-nurse told me that my haemoglobin fell to 7 g/100 ml whereas my normal level is 14 g/100 ml. There were no facilities to give me a blood transfusion which I'm sure they would have done at home. I couldn't feed Benjie because I had no milk.

My periods never came back properly; I had just the odd one, very light, every now and then. Although we take no precautions, I've never become pregnant again. I put on a certain amount of weight and I lost my libido; I just wasn't interested in sex any more. I began to feel tired all the time and lost my sparkle. Also I became constipated which I'd never been before, and when we returned to England, when Benjie was four, I couldn't stand the cold.

I went to my doctor in England and she pointed out that the hair under my arms had disappeared and my pubic hair was very sparse; something I hadn't noticed because it happened so slowly. She quickly confirmed that I was hypothyroid but was surprised that my TSH level was not raised at all. I think it was that which made her realize my pituitary had packed up. She sent me to a specialist who did a lot of tests one morning. He found that my ovaries and my adrenal glands, as well as my thyroid, were not working properly because most of my pituitary had been destroyed when I had that ghastly postpartum haemorrhage. As a result my pituitary no longer produces enough TSH or the other hormones that should activate my ovaries and adrenals.

I'm feeling fine now—better than I have for years. Of course I have to take a lot of pills but I'm used to that and never forget. I take thyroxine for my thyroid, a steroid called hydrocortisone twice a day for my adrenals, and oestrogens—hormone replacement therapy really—for my inactive ovaries.

Silent thyroiditis

This is an uncommon cause of hyperthyroidism. It is called 'silent' because the thyroid gland is not tender as in subacute viral thyroiditis (Chapter 9) nor is it much enlarged.

The exact cause is not known. There is no good evidence of a virus infection and it appears to be due to a short-lived autoimmune disorder, similar but not identical to Hashimoto's thyroiditis. It occurs more often in women than men, and is particularly common in the postpartum period (see p. 143). Perhaps because of greater awareness, silent thyroiditis seems to be more common in certain States in America than it is in Europe. Although it varies from State to State, silent thyroiditis is the cause of hyperthyroidism in some 10 per cent of patients in the USA.

What happens in silent thyroiditis?

If you develop silent thyroiditis you will become thyrotoxic (p. 41) but the degree of this is seldom severe, nor will you have eye complications. The level of thyroid hormones in your blood will be raised and your TSH depressed. However, the most important finding is that a technetium or radio-iodine scan will show a *reduced* uptake of the isotope by your thyroid gland because the thyrotoxicosis is due to the release of pre-formed thyroid hormones stored in the gland. This cardinal difference in radio-isotope uptake distinguishes silent thyroiditis from Graves' disease.

How will I be treated?

Silent thyroiditis is a relatively short-lived condition that remits spontaneously in 2–6 months. If your symptoms are mild, no treatment may be necessary. If they are troublesome, a beta-blocker will prove helpful; if severe, prednisolone is used as in the treatment of viral thyroiditis (p. 108). The more rigorous treatments used for the treatment of Graves' disease (Chapter 4), such as radio-iodine or thyroidectomy, are quite inappropriate for you because after a few months you will get better.

Are there any after-effects?

In about half the patients who have silent thyroiditis, after the hyperthyroidism has remitted and they have become euthyroid, there follows a phase of hypothyroidism. This is most often seen in postpartum women (p. 143). The phase of thyroid deficiency is usually short-lived too, lasting 2–4 months, but in about a quarter of the patients it is permanent and this will necessitate life-long thyroxine replacement treatment.

Thyroid crisis or storm

This is a rare condition in which a patient with thyrotoxicosis has a sudden and severe exacerbation of their hyperthyroid symptoms. This usually comes about as a result of some intercurrent illness such as influenza, a sore throat, or pneumonia in a person who does not know they are thyrotoxic or in a patient whose hyperthyroidism is not being adequately controlled. In the old days a thyroid crisis or storm was not uncommon when surgeons operated on patients who had not been properly prepared by modern methods for the operation and had not been rendered euthyroid. An excess of thyroid hormones was released into the bloodstream as the surgeon handled the incompletely prepared thyroid gland during its subtotal removal.

What happens in a thyroid crisis?

The excess of thyroid hormones in the blood induces a fever, a very rapid heart beat which is often irregular due to atrial fibrillation, cardiac failure, profound sweating with loss of body water, a state of shock with a low blood pressure, and mental confusion or delirium. The outcome may be fatal.

How is a thyroid crisis treated?

The best treatment is prevention, but this is not always possible if the patient does not know or does not show evidence that she is thyrotoxic. If a thyroid storm does occur, treatment with potassium iodide intravenously, propylthiouracil and beta-blockers, as well as replacement of fluid by intravenous infusion must be prompt.

Apathetic hyperthyroidism

This is a very rare and rather mysterious condition that occurs only in elderly patients, whose hyperthyroidism has usually been neglected, undiagnosed, and therefore untreated for several years. The clinical picture is such that apathetic thyrotoxicosis may easily escape recognition because it is so divergent from the familiar clinical picture of hyperthyroidism seen in younger patients.

The patient is emotionally flat and depressed in contrast to the usual picture of anxiety. Instead of being restless the patient with apathetic thyrotoxicosis is lethargic and underactive, and often has a poor appetite. Although there may be a history or evidence of weight loss, the patient appears bloated. Seldom is there marked thyroid enlargement or any eye complications. The pulse may be slow or normal as opposed to the expected increase in rate. Sometimes the illness is mistakenly attributed to the patient getting old, to some hidden cancer, or to clinical depression.

Apathetic hyperthyroidism responds well to antithyroid drugs and sometimes this treatment is continued for many years unless it is more appropriate to induce a permanent cure with radio-iodine.

The 'sick euthyroid' syndrome

This is not really a true thyroid disorder that you need worry about; it is more a problem and matter of concern to your doctor. If you become seriously ill from almost any cause, physical or psychological, the level of total and free T_3 in your blood may drop below normal and in severe cases your total and free T_4 may also become somewhat low. This may suggest to your doctor that you are thyroid deficient, but you are not because the level of TSH in your blood is not raised. As you recover from whatever non-thyroid illness you have, the level of the thyroid hormones returns to normal.

Riedel's thyroiditis

This is an extremely rare condition in which the thyroid gland becomes replaced by scarring fibrous tissue. The thyroid may be tender and feels as hard as wood. Because of this the condition is also known as ligneous (woody) or invasive fibrous thyroiditis.

The gland becomes attached to the overlying skin and to deeper structures in the neck so that your windpipe may be constricted and involvement of the nerves to your vocal cords makes your voice weak or husky. Swallowing may be difficult. Without a biopsy it may be difficult for your doctor to distinguish this condition from an undifferentiated anaplastic cancer (p. 129), and an operation is usually required to relieve the constriction of the windpipe.

Riedel's thyroiditis may be associated with similar fibrotic changes that involve the covering of the intestines (peritoneal fibrosis), structures in the back of your abdomen (retroperitoneal fibrosis), the duct that carries bile from the liver to the intestines (sclerosing cholangitis), or structures in the centre of the chest (mediastinal fibrosis). The cause of this very uncommon condition is unknown.

Suppurative thyroiditis

This too is very uncommon. In suppurative thyroiditis your thyroid gland becomes infected with pus-forming bacteria such as staphylococci which are the cause of boils, or some other micro-organism. Your thyroid gland becomes acutely inflamed and very painful. You will have a high fever and be very ill. The infection may spread to other parts of your body. The response to drainage of a pus-filled abscess and an appropriate antibiotic is usually rapid.

Thyroid hormone resistance

This rare congenital, and sometimes familial, genetic disorder occurs with equal frequency in both sexes. There are mutations in the gene responsible for the thyroid receptors on the cells in your body and the cells fail to respond properly to the thyroid hormones. This results in the body trying to compensate by the thyroid secreting increased amounts of T_4 and T_3. Thus the blood level of these hormones are high although the TSH level is not suppressed. Because the abnormality in the thyroxine receptors may vary from one tissue or organ to another, the responsiveness of the cells to the excess thyroid hormones also varies. Often there is retardation of growth and a delay in the way that the bones mature. Some of the cells in the brain may be relatively unresponsive so that the patient has learning difficulties and an attention deficit with difficulty in concentrating, although the intelligence quotient is usually normal. Other tissues continue to respond to the increased amounts of thyroid hormones and this may be manifest by hyperactivity and a rapid heart rate. About 40 per cent of these patients have a goitre.

The patient may be given triiodothyronine (T_3) which increases the blood level of this hormone even more above the normal level and this may help to surmount the resistance of the tissues.

In the past some patients with thyroid hormone resistance have been mistakenly diagnosed as having hyperthyroidism and been subjected to subtotal thyroidectomy or radio-iodine treatment. This is an understandable mistake when the thyroid hormones are greatly increased and the patient has an increased pulse rate. However, a warning note should have been sounded by finding that the TSH was not suppressed. Those patients, who were operated upon and made worse, need larger than normal replacement therapy to provide higher levels of T_4 and T_3 to surmount the tissue's resistance to the thyroid hormones.

Questions and Answers

Q.1   My grandmother had her thyroid removed for Graves' disease when she was quite young; it must have been in the 1930s. She tells me she had to wait until the winter before they would operate. Why was that, and why do you say I can have my operation later this summer?

A.   In those days it wasn't always easy to control a patient's thyrotoxicosis before surgery was done. Antithyroid drugs and beta-blockers hadn't been invented. Your granny would have been admitted to hospital and given Lugol's iodine for about 10 days. Her pulse, particularly when she was asleep at night, would have been recorded and would be expected to fall to less than 80 beats a minute. She would also be expected to gain some weight before it was safe to operate. It was also found safer to operate in cold weather than in hot. Nowadays we can prepare you much more safely and not do the operation until tests show you're euthyroid.

Q.2   You say my pituitary gland was damaged when I had my postpartum haemorrhage. Will it ever recover?

A.   Sometimes it does if the damage is slight, but your haemorrhage was severe and occurred many years ago. Judging by the present tests, the damage to your pituitary was severe and I'm afraid there is no chance of any recovery now.

Q.3   You say I've got hypopituitarism but my GP says I've got Sheehan's syndrome. Who is right?

A.   They're one and the same thing when the pituitary has been damaged as a result of a haemorrhage associated with childbirth. The late Professor Sheehan of Liverpool first clearly described the association.

Q.4   Have I got to take all these tablets for the rest of my life?

A.   Yes, for the rest of your life, although when you're about 65 or 70 we may stop the female hormone tablets—perhaps earlier. They won't cost you anything in the British National Health Service because currently medicines for an endocrine deficiency are dispensed free of cost to the patient. In any case, these are not as expensive as you might think, but they are essential for your continued well-being.

Q.5.   I had hypothyroidism about 2 months after my son was born. They gave me thyroxine for a couple of months and I got better quite quickly. The thyroxine was stopped and I'm fine now. When I have my next child is the same thing going to happen again?

A.   It is likely to. Before you had your son they found at the antenatal clinic that you had thyroid autoantibodies to thyroglobulin and thyroid peroxidase—TPO antibodies—in your blood. This is often a forewarning that you may have either hyper- or hypothyroidism, sometimes one after the other, during the first 3–6 months after delivery. This is exactly what happened to you. You still have these antibodies which are causing no trouble now but when you become pregnant next time, the whole thing may well happen again.

15

Other diseases associated with thyroid disorders

Autoimmune diseases

Certain people and certain families are more prone to autoimmune diseases than others, and hence other auto-immune diseases are associated with thyroid autoimmune disorders. For example, if you develop Hashimoto's thyr-oiditis you may find that your grandmother had Graves' hyperthyroidism. In other words two different types of autoimmune thyroid disease are occurring in the same family but skipping a generation, as often happens. Autoimmune thyroid diseases certainly run in families as do other autoimmune disorders, although not all members of a family are so affected. There are several other auto-immune diseases that you should know about, because a relative of yours may have got one or you, already with an autoimmune thyroid disease, could possibly one day develop a non-thyroid autoimmune disorder, uncommon though this may be.

The following are autoimmune disorders that may some-times be associated with autoimmune thyroid disease.

Addisonian (pernicious) anaemia

This is a particular type of anaemia which should no longer be called 'pernicious' because it is so easily treated. In Addisonian anaemia (named after the physician at Guy's Hospital who first described it in 1855), the body makes antibodies against certain cells in the wall of the stomach.

These cells secrete a substance, intrinsic factor, which promotes the absorption of vitamin B_{12} from the intestinal tract and this is essential for the making of red blood corpuscles. Addisonian anaemia is easily corrected by giving injections of vitamin B_{12} every 6 weeks or so.

Diabetes mellitus

Sugar diabetes, particularly the type that starts in young people and requires insulin for its control, occurs with an increased incidence in the families of patients who have autoimmune thyroid diseases. Diabetes mellitus is at least in part an autoimmune disease caused by antibodies attacking the cells in the pancreas that secrete the hormone insulin. The presenting symptoms of juvenile or insulin-dependent diabetes, which may come on quite suddenly, are the passing of large volumes of urine, increased thirst, tiredness, and weight loss. Treatment is by diet and injections of insulin.

Addison's disease of the adrenal glands

Lying just above the kidneys are two small endocrine glands—the adrenal or suprarenal glands—which secrete steroid hormones such as cortisone. These hormones are essential to life and regulate the blood pressure and the response to infections, stress, physical accidents, and surgery. Failure of the adrenal glands was described by the same physician, Dr Addison, who described pernicious anaemia. The adrenal glands may be destroyed by tuberculosis but nowadays the most common cause is autoimmune destruction of the adrenal cells. Addison's adrenal failure is characterized by extreme weakness and fatigue, a low blood pressure, and darkening of the skin, particularly over the knuckles and of the mucous membrane inside the mouth. It responds well to replacement therapy with cortisone and related steroids taken by mouth. When a patient with Hashimoto's thyroiditis also develops Addison's adrenal failure, the condition is known as Schmidt's syndrome. It is important that the adrenal insufficiency component is treated with steroids before thyroxine is started because if thyroxine is given first, the adrenal insufficiency will be made worse, sometimes dangerously so.

Polymyalgia rheumatica and giant-cell arteritis

These two diseases are related. The first is characterized by pains in the muscles and joints. Giant-cell arteritis, or cranial arteritis as it is also called, gives rise to headaches, fever, and general malaise. Treatment for either condition is with corticosteroids in carefully controlled doses. Either or both may occasionally be associated with hypothyroidism caused by Hashimoto's thyroiditis and may occur before or after the thyroid deficiency declares itself.

Vitiligo

This is a skin disorder, also known as leucoderma (white skin), in which patches of white skin devoid of normal pigment develop. Vitiligo is a common associate of all autoimmune diseases and may be looked upon as a 'marker' or an indicator for some autoimmune disorder that may develop in the distant future.

Alopecia and hair loss

Alopecia is an autoimmune disease that causes patchy loss of hair, usually on the scalp but sometimes in the beard area. The areas of hair loss may be small and few, or they may be quite large.

Generalized loss of hair, particularly from the scalp, also occurs in patients with hyper- or hypothyroidism. There is some evidence that antithyroid drugs used for the treatment of hyperthyroidism may also increase the loss of scalp hair. Recovery of the lost hair is always slow after the underlying condition is treated, but usually the outcome is satisfactory.

Myasthenia gravis

This rare muscle disorder caused by an autoimmune disturbance is said to be more common in patients with

Graves' disease than in the general population. Often it first affects the muscles of the eyes and leads to double vision. Later other muscles in the limbs or trunk may become involved. As the day progresses the patient experiences increasing weakness, and the more you try to do the weaker and more tired you become. There may be difficulty in swallowing, the voice becomes nasal and breathing may become a struggle. The response to treatment is usually satisfactory.

Let one of our patients tell her story. She started with Graves' disease; then developed diabetes, only later to have Addisonian anaemia associated with vitiligo and ended up with hypothyroidism due to Hashimoto's disease:

I'm now aged 55. I trained as a lawyer but all my working life I've been in local government. At the age of 12, I developed Graves' disease. I remember eating like a horse, but despite this I lost a lot of weight. My eyes became slightly starey. I was very clumsy and was always dropping things. My overactive thyroid was brought under control with antithyroid tablets, and everything was all right until, at the age of 17, I began to lose weight again. I was very thirsty and used to take a jug of water to bed with me. My sleep was disturbed by having to get up several times at night to pass urine. Our doctor found I'd developed diabetes, and this was treated with diet and twice-daily insulin injections which I soon got used to. When I was 30 I was made deputy head of my department. Normally I'm pretty lively, but I became tired and my aunt commented on how pale I'd become. I'd also developed some funny white patches on my forearms. The doctor at the hospital where I go for my diabetes found I'd developed Addisonian anaemia. This quickly responded to injections of vitamin B_{12} which I was given by our family doctor but I could have given them to myself as I'm used to injecting myself with insulin. I remained very well until I was aged about 45 when I began to feel the cold terribly and used to complain to the engineer at the Town Hall where I worked about the temperature in my office. He took no notice of me and I wore thicker clothes in a vain attempt to keep warm. Not until the next winter did I mention this to my family doctor and he spotted that I'd become thyroid deficient. Apparently I'd developed another sort of thyroid trouble called Hashimoto's thyroiditis but there was no swelling in my neck like there was when I had Graves' disease. The hypothyroidism was put right by giving me thyroxine. I feel fine now. I take my thyroxine tablets every day, have my vitamin injection every month, and give myself insulin injections twice daily.

Now you will understand why your doctor may do tests unrelated to your thyroid condition to be sure you have not got some other incipient autoimmune disorder, such as Addisonian anaemia, which may declare itself later on in your life.

Psychological problems

Stress

Many patients ask whether stress is the cause of thyroid disorders because they note that the onset of Grave's disease, in particular, often seems to occur following some major stress, such as bereavement, loss of a job, an accident, or some other major psychological upset. This association has also been noted in patients who develop hypothyroidism caused by Hashimoto's thyroiditis.

There is evidence that stress is not the *primary* cause of such autoimmune disorders. During the Nazi occupation of Belgium in the Second World War, for example, there was no increase in the incidence of Graves' disease in Brussels despite oppression, fear, deprivation, and malnutrition. Equally, in Northern Ireland during the troubles that have afflicted that country since 1968 there has been no increase in the incidence of Graves' disease. The problem is, of course, that different psychological disturbances affect different people in different ways. A sudden unexpected bereavement may have a greater impact than an anticipated death. Psychological disturbances can certainly influence the immune system and current evidence suggests that stress may aggravate a pre-existing auto-immune disorder, inducing hyper- or hypothyroidism only in those with the genetic make-up that makes them susceptible to a pre-existing but subclinical autoimmune disease.

Anxiety state

Most patients with Graves' disease admit to being anxious. Indeed anxiety is a prominent feature in many patients with this condition. They have a fast pulse rate, a tremor, are conscious of the beating of their heart, and they sweat excessively. In addition they are anxious about what normally would be everyday events. They worry about everything—whether the children will come home from school safely, whether their spouse will have a car accident, or whether the boiler will go wrong. This anxiety state usually remits when the hyperthyroidism is treated, but in some patients it persists in lesser degree. This is a psychological disturbance, whether the patient concedes this or not, and usually she does. The anxiety often responds to treatment with a beta-blocker but sometimes other drugs have to be used.

Clinical depression

The association between hypothyroidism and clinical depression has been recognized for many years. Many patients with thyroid deficiency feel 'low'. They find life unenjoyable; they worry and are gloomy. At night they do not sleep well, waking up soon after they get to sleep. They feel exhausted in the morning and do not want to get up. They just feel tired and 'awful'. This clinical depression often remits when the hypothyroidism is corrected, but in some patients, despite the correct replacement dosage of thyroxine for several months, it persists.

The depression is due to a disturbance in the chemicals, the neurotransmitters, that regulate the cells in the brain. It is not due to 'lack of moral fibre' as some patients may mistakenly think. Persistent depression after correction of thyroid deficiency is quite common and is a cause for patients being dissatisfied with their response to thyroxine treatment. It is, of course, essential that the correct replacement is being given and most patients with thyroid deficiency feel at their best when the dosage of thyroxine raises their free thyroxine level towards the upper end of the normal range, or even a little above it. This may reduce the thyroid stimulating hormone (TSH) level towards the bottom of the normal range or even a little below it, but not so low as to be undetectable. If you have received for several months the amount of thyroxine that meets these criteria but still continue to feel generally unwell, it is likely that your ill-health is due to a persistent degree of clinical depression which merits treatment in its own right. Fortunately there are many psychotropic drugs, with few side-effects, that will correct this situation.

Atrial fibrillation

An irregular, and often fast, beating of the heart, called atrial fibrillation, is common in elderly patients with hyperthyroidism. There are many other causes of atrial fibrillation—the most common being ischaemic heart disease (coronary artery disease)—but the more easily treated hyperthyroidism may be missed if the symptoms and signs of hyperthyroidism are not prominent, as often happens in older patients. Thus cardiologists usually check the thyroid hormones and TSH levels in any patient who develops atrial fibrillation. In thyrotoxicosis, correction of the atrial fibrillation often occurs spontaneously when the thyroid overactivity is brought under control. If it is not, further measures may be required to slow the irregular heart or convert the rhythm to a normal, regular one.

Dyslexia

It appears that dyslexia is more common in families with autoimmune thyroid disease than in the population at large. Children with dyslexia show a delay in their ability to read and later have difficulty with spelling and writing. These children are by no means stupid and often are very bright but because of their handicap they may fall behind at school. Boys are more often affected than girls and they tend to be left-handed.

Questions and Answers

Q.1   Are these other autoimmune diseases common in patients like me with thyroid disease? How likely am I to get one?

A.   They are more common than in the general population but it is difficult to give you precise figures. All of us have had experience of the occasional patient with autoimmune thyroid disease of one sort or another who, for example, has developed pernicious anaemia later in life.

Q.2   My grandmother says she had myxoedema 20 years ago; she's on thyroxine. Now you tell me I've got an overactive thyroid gland. Is there any connection?

A.   Yes, there is. Your grandmother and you both have autoimmune thyroid diseases of different kinds, and this does tend to run in families.

Q.3   I've Hashimoto's thyroiditis for years and now you tell me I've got Addisonian anaemia. What is going to happen to me next?

A.   Nothing more I hope, but we should keep a regular eye on you in the remote possibility of yet another autoimmune disease developing.

Glossary of terms

Addisonian anaemia: a type of anaemia, also known as pernicious anaemia before effective treatment became available, caused by an autoimmune disorder which prevents absorption of vitamin B_{12} from the intestine and may be associated with Hashimoto's thyroiditis (see vitamin B_{12} below).

Addison's disease: this disease is the consequence of failure of the adrenal glands, usually caused by an autoimmune disorder. It may be associated with Hashimoto's thyroiditis.

Adrenal glands: two small endocrine glands that lie on top of your kidneys and secrete cortisone-like steroid hormones. Normal function is essential to life.

Agranulocytosis: a disappearance of granulocytes (neutrophil white corpuscles) from the peripheral blood. This opens the door and renders you liable to any intercurrent infection. Agranulocytosis may rarely occur as a side-effect of treatment with antithyroid drugs but also occurs with several other types of medicine.

Anaplastic: a word used to describe very undifferentiated cancer cells which are aggressively malignant.

Antibodies: chemicals (proteins) that are formed in the body by lymphocytes (a particular type of white corpuscle in the blood) in response to invasion by any foreign protein (antigen). Such antibodies constitute a defence against viruses and bacteria that you may encounter during your life. Autoantibodies are antibodies that react against certain of your own tissues, such as your thyroid cells.

Autoantibodies against 'self' (your own cells) are important in the causation of Graves' disease and Hashimoto's thyroiditis, and many other autoimmune disorders.

Antithyroid drugs: these drugs, such as carbimazole, methimazole and propylthiouracil, suppress hormone manufacture by the cells of your thyroid gland.

Apathetic hyperthyroidism: an uncommon form of hyperthyroidism usually seen only in old people.

Atrophic: destruction of a tissue or an organ which becomes wasted and fibrosed (scar tissue). This is seen in atrophic hypothyroidism.

Autoimmune disease: a disease that results from the body making antibodies which attack normal cells or tissues in your body. There are many autoimmune diseases, such as Hashimoto's thyroiditis, pernicious anaemia, Addisonian adrenal insufficiency, and others.

Benign: not malignant or cancerous.

Beta-adrenergic blocking drugs: these slow the heart rate, reduce palpitations and sweating, and improve some of the other features of thyroid overactivity, but do not cure the underlying disease.

Beta-blockers: a colloquial name for beta-adrenergic blocking drugs, such as propranolol.

Biopsy: a term used to describe removal of a small piece of tissue in order to examine it under the microscope. A biopsy of the thyroid gland may be made with little discomfort by a fine-needle aspiration or during a surgical operation.

Calcitonin: a hormone secreted by the medullary, C-, or parafollicular cells that reside in the thyroid gland but are not of thyroid origin. Calcitonin influences the calcium level in your blood and the amount of calcium in your bones. Measurement of the calcitonin level can be used as a marker to assess the effectiveness of treatment of a medullary cell carcinoma.

Carbimazole: a commonly used antithyroid drug.

Carcinoma: cancer. A differentiated carcinoma of the thyroid gland is one of the malignant diseases that is most amendable to treatment. An undifferentiated (anaplastic) carcinoma is more invasive.

Carrier proteins: substances to which the thyroid hormones are loosely attached as they are transported round the body in the bloodstream (see thyroxine-binding globulin).

CAT or CT scan: computer assisted tomography is a special type of X-ray examination, used in thyroid disorders to examine particularly the eye changes in Graves' disease and sometimes a retrosternal goitre, and compression or displacement of the windpipe.

Cholesterol: a particular type of fat found in the bloodstream. The level may be raised in hypothyroidism and decreased in hyperthyroidism, but it is also affected by many other factors.

Chronic lymphocytic goitre: another name for Hashimoto's thyroiditis.

'Cold' nodule: a nodule in the thyroid gland that does not take up a radio-isotope such as technetium or radio-iodine.

Congenital: existing at birth. A baby may be born with congenital hypothyroidism.

Corticosteroids: also called 'steroids', are cortisone-like hormones secreted by the adrenal (suprarenal) glands and as drugs are used to suppress an autoimmune response.

Cortisone: a corticosteroid drug now largely replaced by prednisone, prednisolone, or methylprednisolone.

Cretinism: thyroid deficiency occurring in an infant or child and associated with impaired mental development.

CT scan: see CAT scan.

Cyst: a hollow tumour, usually benign, which may contain fluid.

Decompression: surgical decompression of the bony orbits, in which the eyes lie, may be necessary to reduce the intra-orbital pressure in severe ophthalmopathy.

De Quervain's thyroiditis: the same as subacute viral thyroiditis.

Diffuse toxic goitre: another name for Graves' or von Basedow's disease. 'Diffuse' because the whole gland is generally enlarged and 'toxic' because excess secretion of the thyroid hormones induces thyrotoxicosis.

Diplopia: double vision as may occur in Graves' ophthalmopathy.

Dyshormonogenesis: a defect in one or more of the several chemical steps that take place in the manufacture of thyroid hormones. The defect varies in severity and may be a rare cause of thyroid underactivity and/or a goitre in infancy or childhood.

Dyslexia: a disorder of reading and writing that may occur in children.

Endemic goitre: when more than 20 per cent of a population being surveyed are found to have a goitre, the goitre is said to be endemic.

Endocrine gland: a gland that forms a hormone which it secretes into the bloodstream. These chemical messengers affect cells and tissues far removed from where they are produced.

Erythrocyte sedimentation rate (ESR): this is a non-specific test to see if a patient is ill, usually as the result of some infection. The rate at which the red cells in the blood (the red corpuscles or erythrocytes) sink or sediment in a special long glass tube filled with blood is measured over a period of 1 hour. The result is expressed as the distance the red cells fall, measured in millimetres (mm) per hour.

Euthyroid: this means that you have normal levels of thyroid hormones in your blood. You do not have over- or underactivity of your thyroid gland.

Exophthalmometer: an instrument for measuring the degree of protrusion of your eyeballs.

Exophthalmos: also known as proptosis. This means a protrusion of the eyeballs which are pushed forwards. A feature of Graves' ophthalmopathy.

Fibrosis: the deposition of fibrous connective tissue (scarring) in an organ that has been subjected to injury, usually inflammation, as may occur in the thyroid gland late in the course of Hashimoto's thyroiditis.

Free thyroxine index: this is not really a test in its own right. It is a mathematical calculation derived from the total thyroxine level and the T_3-resin-binding test. It makes allowance for alterations, upwards or downwards, in the proteins that carry your thyroxine and reflects indirectly the amount of thyroxine which is unattached to protein and floating free in the water of the blood. This 'test' has largely been replaced, and rightly so, by the measurement of the free thyroid hormones, the free T_4 and the free T_3 (see below).

Free thyroxine (T_4) level: this test measures the tiny amount of thyroxine that is present in the water of the blood, and which is a fraction of the very much larger amount that is loosely bound to the thyroxine-binding carrier proteins. The advantage of measuring the unbound 'free' thyroxine is that the level is less influenced by changes in the amount of the transport proteins. It is this free thyroxine that determines your thyroid status. For this reason in many centres measurement of the free thyroxine is now used as a first-line test of thyroid function in preference to the total thyroxine. The normal reference range for the free T_4 will depend on the exact technique used but, in round figures, is usually about 9 to about 25 picomoles per litre (pmol/L). Levels greater than 26 pmol/L occur in most cases of hyperthyroidism, and below 8 pmol/L in thyroid deficiency. The more severe the thyrotoxicosis the higher will be the free T_4 level and the more severe the hypothyroidism the lower the free T_4.

Occasionally the free T_4 test gives misleading results if certain interfering antibodies or an unusual albumin carrier protein is present in your blood. Low levels may sometimes occur in a variety of non-thyroidal illnesses (see 'sick euthyroid' syndrome).

Free triiodothyronine (T_3) level: this test measures the level of unbound 'free' T_3 in your blood. In normal people the reference range is of the order of about 3 to about 9 pmol/L but varies slightly according to the technique used. The free T_3 is particularly useful in the diagnosis of hyperthyroidism because it may rise, some weeks or months, before the free thyroxine (fT_4) level does. Indeed, there are some patients with thyrotoxicosis who never develop a raised thyroxine level (so-called T_3-toxicosis). The free T_3 is less useful than the free T_4 in diagnosing hypothyroidism, because the failing thyroid gland finds it easier to produce triiodothyronine and the level of T_3 falls later than does the T_4 level. Low free T_3 levels are common in patients suffering from any non-thyroidal physical or psychiatric disease (see 'sick euthyroid' syndrome).

Goitre: any enlargement of the thyroid gland is called a goitre. The word is spelt goiter in the United States.

Graves' disease: an autoimmune disorder of the thyroid gland, named after the Irish physician who described it, that causes overactivity and increased levels of T_4 and/or T_3 in the blood (see also Von Basedow's disease).

Hashimoto's thyroiditis: an autoimmune disorder of the thyroid gland, named after the Japanese surgeon who first described it, which may induce thyroid enlargement (a goitre) and later causes underactivity of the gland (hypothyroidism).

Hashitoxicosis: a temporary episode of hyperthyroidism in a patient with Hashimoto's thyroiditis.

Hormone: a chemical substance, made in an endocrine gland, that is secreted into the bloodstream and affects tissues elsewhere in the body.

Hormone replacement therapy (HRT): this is the use of a hormone given to treat a condition in which the naturally secreted hormone is deficient. However, HRT is usually used to describe the administration of ovarian hormones (oestrogens) to women at the time surrounding their menopause.

'Hot' nodule: a nodule in the thyroid gland that actively takes up a tracer dose of a radio-isotope to a greater degree than does the surrounding normal thyroid tissue.

Hyperthyroidism: overactivity of the thyroid gland, which is characterized by certain symptoms and signs, a raised level of T_4 and/or T_3 and usually a suppressed TSH level in the blood.

Hypopituitarism: underactivity of the pituitary gland. This may reduce just one, several, or all the different hormones secreted by the gland, including the thyroid-stimulating hormone (TSH).

Hypothalamus: the hypothalamus is a small neuroendocrine gland located in the brain close to the pituitary. It secretes a number of different hormones. One of these is the thyrotrophin-releasing hormone (TRH) which stimulates the TSH-secreting cells in the pituitary.

Hypothyroidism: a condition in which the thyroid gland fails to secrete enough hormones.

Iodine: this element is an essential constituent of the thyroid hormones and is obtained from your diet. It is present in iodized salt, sea-fish, milk and other dairy products, and some vegetables. In certain parts of the world iodine is present in too small quantities so that the thyroid gland in the inhabitants, particularly women, is liable to become enlarged (endemic goitre) and the women may become hypothyroid.

Isotope: the form of an element with a slightly different atomic weight but the same chemical properties. Radioactive isotopes of iodine and technetium are used in the diagnosis of thyroid disorders and radio-iodine also in the treatment of some thyroid conditions.

Isthmus: this is the little bridge of thyroid tissue across the trachea (windpipe) that connects the left and right lobes of your thyroid gland.

Kelp: this is a 'health' food product derived from seaweed and contains much iodine.

Lymphadenoid goitre: the same as nodular enlargement of the thyroid, as in Hashimoto's thyroiditis.

Lymph gland (lymph node): a small gland that 'filters' lymph and when enlarged is most easily felt in the neck, under the arms, or in the groin. Enlargement of a lymph node in the neck is most often the consequence of pharyngitis (a 'sore-throat') but may be related to thyroid disease.

Lymphocyte: a particular type of white corpuscle that is concerned with the recognition of foreign proteins and the manufacture of antibodies.

Lymphoma: a malignant tumour of the lymphocytes that may involve the thyroid gland.

Medullary cell cancer: a cancer of the medullary, C-, or parafollicular cells that lodge in the thyroid gland and secrete the hormone calcitonin.

Metastases: a secondary deposit of cancer cells at a site distant from the original or primary cancer.

Methimazole: an antithyroid drug commonly used in the United States.

Microsomal antibodies: various techniques of increasing sensitivity (precipitin, latex, tanned red cells agglutination, enzyme-linked immunosorbent tests) are used to identify and quantify these antibodies. Microsomal, also known as thyroid peroxidase (TPO), antibodies are cytotoxic, which means that they act against the thyroid cells and destroy them. They are present in most patients with Hashimoto's thyroiditis and also in some with Graves' disease.

Multinodular goitre: a goitre that contains many nodules. If you have a multinodular goitre you may be euthyroid now but later in life you may become hyperthyroid or hypothyroid.

Myxoedema: an advanced form of hypothyroidism. The term, strictly speaking, applies to the thickened skin which is characteristic of severe thyroid deficiency.

Neonatal: the first 4 weeks of a baby's life.

Neutrophil: a white corpuscle that very rarely is reduced in numbers as a side-effect of antithyroid drug treatment (see agranulocytosis).

Nodule: a lump in the thyroid gland.

Oculomotor muscles: these muscles control the movements of your eyeballs. They may become affected in Graves' ophthalmopathy so that you have difficulty in looking up or you may see double when you look to one side or the other.

Oestrogens: female ovarian hormones. Among their many other actions they increase the level of the thyroxine-binding proteins that carry thyroxine and T_3 in your bloodstream. When increased, as in pregnancy or if you are taking an oestrogen-containing oral contraceptive 'pill', they cause elevation of the total, but not the free, thyroid hormones.

Ophthalmopathy: this comprises a variety of changes in

the eyes that occur characteristically in many patients with Graves' disease.

Ophthalmoplegia: this term is used to describe weakness or paralysis of the oculomotor muscles that move the eyeballs. Ophthalmoplegia may cause double vision (diplopia).

Orbit: the rigid bony socket in which the eye lies.

Osteoporosis: a thinning of the bones that occurs in women particularly at the time of the menopause and in men as they grow older. It is aggravated by hyperthyroidism.

Parathyroid glands: four little glands close to the thyroid that secrete the parathyroid hormone which controls the level of calcium in your blood.

Pendred's syndrome: the association of infantile hypothyroidism and deafness.

Pernicious anaemia: see Addisonian anaemia. 'Pernicious' is not a good word because the condition is easily treated.

Phaeochromocytoma: a tumour of the adrenal gland(s) that secretes hormones that affect your blood pressure, usually causing high blood pressure (hypertension).

Pituitary gland: an endocrine gland in the base of the skull that secretes a large number of different hormones. Of particular interest in thyroid disorders is the thyroid-stimulating hormone (TSH), also known as thyrotrophin.

Plummer's disease: named after the American physician who described it, is another name for a toxic multinodular goitre.

Postpartum: after delivery of a baby.

Pretibial myxoedema: a skin condition affecting usually the lower legs and feet. It is associated with Graves' disease in some patients. The term is misleading because it has nothing to do with *hypo*thyroidism.

Proptosis: protrusion of the eyes. The same as exophthalmos.

Propylthiouracil: an antithyroid drug.

Radio-iodine: there are three different radio-active isotopes of iodine which may be used in the diagnosis of thyroid disorders. One isotope, ^{131}I, is also used for the treatment of hyperthyroidism, thyroid cancer, and other thyroid disorders. The isotopes with a shorter duration of action (half-life), ^{123}I and ^{132}I, may be used for diagnostic tests.

Recurrent laryngeal nerves: these are the two nerves that supply your vocal cords. They may be injured during thyroid surgery or involved by thyroid cancer. This causes huskiness of the voice.

Reflexes: the tendon reflexes, tested by your doctor tapping, for example, the tendon just below your knee-cap or the Achilles tendon at your heel, may be slow to relax in hypothyroidism and be unusually brisk in hyperthyroidism.

Replacement therapy: this is the use of a hormone given by your doctor to make good the deficient secretion of one of your endocrine glands.

Reverse T_3: a biologically inactive form of T_3 which is formed from normally active T_3 and has the same atomic constituents but the molecule is the mirror image of normal T_3.

Riedel's thyroiditis: a very rare form of hardening of the thyroid gland due to fibrous tissue.

Scan: an examination by X-rays (CAT or CT scan), by ultrasound (echo- or sonogram), by magnetic resonance imaging (MRI), or by radio-isotopes (scintigram), which produces what amounts to three-dimensional pictures of the organ being studied.

Sheehan's syndrome: hypopituitarism caused by severe loss of blood during or immediately after childbirth. Hypothyroidism is one component of the resulting hormone deficiencies.

Sick euthyroid syndrome: this is a situation in which the patient is suffering from some severe non-thyroid illness and is found to have a depressed blood level of T_3, and sometimes also of T_4. In fact the patient is euthyroid and the TSH level is not raised. As recovery takes place the thyroid function tests return to normal.

Silent thyroiditis: an episode of usually mild and temporary hyperthyroidism due to an autoimmune disorder unaccompanied by any pain or discomfort in the thyroid gland. It is important that this is distinguished from Graves' disease by an isotope scan, which in silent thyroiditis will show reduced uptake, indicating that the gland is putting out but not making too much hormone. The distinction is important because the treatment is so different.

Stridor: a crowing noise made on breathing, usually when asleep, due to many causes but in the context of thyroid disease to compression or displacement of the windpipe (trachea) by a goitre.

Subacute viral thyroiditis: this is the same as viral thyroiditis or de Quervain's disease.

Suppurative thyroiditis: an acute infection of the thyroid gland by micro-organisms that cause the formation of pus.

T_3-toxicosis: a state hyperthyroidism caused by increased secretion of triiodothyronine (T_3) unassociated with an increased blood level of T_4. The TSH level is suppressed. It may occur early in the course of Graves' disease or in association with a 'hot' nodule in the thyroid gland.

Technetium: ^{99m}Tc, or more correctly 99m-technetium pertechnetate, is a radio-isotope with a short half-life that is used for thyroid scintiscans. Throughout this book technetium is used as an abbreviation for technetium pertechnetate.

Tetany: a condition due to a low calcium level in your blood that causes a curious numb feeling round your mouth and induces spasm in the muscles of your hands, and sometimes your feet. It may occur from temporary or permanent damage to your parathyroid glands during thyroid surgery.

Thymus: a gland in the upper chest behind the breastbone that makes certain white corpuscles and is involved in autoimmune processes.

Thyroglobulin: a protein to which the thyroid hormones are attached when they are stored in the thyroid gland. Measurement of the blood level of thyroglobulin is valuable for telling that no normal or malignant thyroid cells are left after total removal of the thyroid gland and/or an ablative therapeutic dose of radio-iodine has been given for the treatment of thyroid cancer. This test is also used for detecting whether any metastases have developed.

Thyroglobulin antibodies: thyroglobulin antibodies are mainly directed against the thyroglobulin stored in the thyroid gland. Increased amounts are usually found in patients with Hashimoto's disease but the microsomal (TPO) antibodies are usually more sensitive in establishing the diagnosis.

Thyroglossal duct: this is a remnant left behind as the thyroid gland descends from its origin at the base of the tongue to the neck in the unborn baby. It may become the site of a thyroglossal cyst.

Thyroid crisis or storm: an acute exacerbation of severe thyrotoxicosis that may be fatal unless treated promptly.

Thyroidectomy: this is the technical term for surgical removal of the thyroid gland. The surgeon may remove all of the gland (total thyroidectomy); the majority, such as seven-eighths (subtotal thyroidectomy); or only a lobe (thyroid lobectomy or hemithyroidectomy).

Thyroiditis: this is an inflammatory condition of the thyroid gland that is usually caused by an autoimmune process (Hashimoto's thyroiditis) or by a virus (subacute viral or de Quervain's thyroiditis). There are other forms of thyroiditis (see also 'silent thyroiditis').

Thyroid-stimulating antibodies and immunoglobulins: these antibodies, also known as thyrotrophin-receptor stimulating antibodies or thyroid-stimulating immunoglobulins, occupy the TSH-receptor sites on the surface of thyroid cells and stimulate the cells to increase their secretion of thyroid hormones. They are the cause of auto-immune hyperthyroidism (Graves' disease). These thyroid stimulating immunoglobulins can be detected in more than 90 per cent of patients with Graves' disease and also occur in 60 per cent of euthyroid patients who have ophthalmic Graves' disease. The same antibody occurs temporarily in some patients with Hashimoto's disease who have a transient episode of hyperthyroidism ('Hashitoxicosis').

Thyroid-stimulating hormone (TSH): this is the hormone secreted by the pituitary gland that regulates the hormonal output from the thyroid gland. Its measurement is used to confirm the diagnosis of hypothyroidism (raised

TSH level) and of hyperthyroidism (depressed TSH level). A low TSH level may also occur under a number of other circumstances:

- during the first 3 months of pregnancy in normal women;

- in some patients with eye symptoms indicative of Graves' ophthalmopathy before hyperthyroidism develops, and in those in whom hyperthyroidism may never develop (ophthalmic Graves' disease);

- in patients who are in remission from, or have been cured of, Graves' disease. This happens because recovery of the previously suppressed pituitary is often delayed for many months;

- in euthyroid patients who have an autonomous nodule or nodules in their thyroid gland;

- in patients with failure of the pituitary gland; and

- in any patient, but particularly the elderly, the secretion of TSH may be temporarily reduced by non-thyroidal illnesses, either physical or psychiatric.

Thyrotoxicosis: another name for hyperthyroidism or thyroid overactivity.

Thyrotoxicosis factitia: the occurrence of hyperthyroidism in a patient who is taking, sometimes undeclared to the doctor, excessive amounts of T_4 or T_3.

Thyrotrophin-releasing hormone (TRH): this hormone is secreted by the hypothalamus and increases the activity of the cells in the pituitary that secrete thyroid-stimulating hormone (TSH).

Thyrotrophin-releasing hormone (TRH) test: injection of synthetic TRH produces a rise of TSH in the blood which, in a normal person, peaks 20 minutes later. This response is absent in thyrotoxic patients and is exaggerated in those with primary hypothyroidism. This forms the basis of the TRH test which is seldom used nowadays because the sensitive TSH assay reliably measures reduced levels of the thyroid-stimulating hormone in hyperthyroidism and increased levels in hypothyroidism.

Thyroxine: one of the thyroid hormones, which contains four iodine atoms and is often called T_4.

Thyroxine-binding globulin (TBG): three main classes of protein carry thyroxine in the bloodstream—globulin, pre-albumin, and albumin. The most important of these is globulin which carries about 70 per cent of the thyroxine. An abnormally low, even absent, or an abnormally high level of thyroxine-binding globulin level may occur as an innocent hereditary abnormality, usually in men. When the TBG is low, the levels of total T_4 and total T_3 are also low, because their main carrier protein is reduced; when the TBG is high, the level of the thyroid hormones is raised, but in both situations the patient is euthyroid and has a normal TSH level and usually normal free T_4 and free T_3 levels.

Total serum thyroxine (T_4) level: this test, which is done on a small sample of blood removed from a vein, measures the total amount of thyroxine per unit of blood and this comprises the T_4 bound to the various different proteins that carry most of the thyroxine. The result may be expressed in terms of the weight of thyroxine per 100 ml of blood (micrograms/100 ml or µg/100 ml) or in terms of the number of molecules of thyroxine per litre (nanomoles/L or nmol/L). The normal reference ranges may differ slightly from one laboratory to another, depending on the exact chemicals (reagents) used and the population of 'healthy' people from whose results the normal range has been derived. In most instances of hyperthyroidism, except of course T_3-toxicosis, the result of the T_4 estimation is unequivocally raised, and in patients with hypothyroidism it is reduced.

The main snag about measuring the total serum T_4 level is that the result depends on the amount of thyroxine bound to the transport proteins. It is the tiny amount of thyroxine which is unbound and floating free in the water of the blood, the free T_4, that determines your thyroid status. Thus the result of the total thyroxine assay is influenced by two factors—the amount of T_4 present, and the amount and the binding capacity of the different carrier proteins.

Table 5   Situations that increase or decrease the level of carrier proteins or otherwise influence the levels of total T_4 and/or total T_3

Increased total T_4 and/or total T_3 levels may occur in:
- Pregnancy

- Oestrogen therapy

- The oral contraceptive pill

- Drug therapy with amiodarone, clofibrate, or phenothiazines (e.g. chlorpromazine)

- Hereditary increased thyroxine-binding globulin

Decreased total T_4 and/or total T_3 levels may occur in:
- Kidney diseases or other causes of low plasma proteins

- Acromegaly (increased growth hormone secretion)

- Cushing's syndrome (hyperadrenocorticism)

- Hereditary low or absent thyroxine-binding globulin

- Andogenic, anabolic, or corticosteroid therapy

- Fenclofenac (Flenac) therapy

- Phenylbutazone (Butacote) therapy

- Phenytoin (Epanutin, Dilantin) therapy

- Salicylate (aspirin) therapy

- Antidepressive therapy

Under certain circumstances, for example in pregnancy, if you are taking the contraceptive pill containing oestrogens, or you are having hormone replacement therapy (HRT) during the menopause, the amount of carrier proteins is increased. This increases the total T_4 level but does not make you hyperthyroid because the free non-protein-bound thyroxine remains normal. Certain drugs, such as aspirin and many others, may occupy the binding sites on the carrier proteins normally reserved for thyroxine. These drugs will therefore tend to lower the total T_4 level by displacing the protein-bound thyroxine.

Because variations in the amount of the carrier proteins and in the number of their binding sites may be induced by hormones, drugs, many non-thyroid diseases, and by genetic factors, most physicians nowadays prefer to measure the free T_4.

Total serum triiodothyronine (T_3) level: this measure of the total serum protein-bound concentration of T_3 has the same disadvantages as measuring the total serum T_4 level. Usually the total T_3 and T_4 levels move in parallel because about one-third of the T_3 is secreted by the thyroid gland and two-thirds is derived in peripheral tissues from the conversion of T_4 to T_3. In T_3-toxicosis the total T_3 is raised but the total T_4 is normal; similarly the free T_3 is raised and the free T_4 is normal. In hypothyroidism the T_3 level is often normal or much less depressed than the T_4 level which is a better indicator of thyroid deficiency, but the TSH level is the best and an even more sensitive test.

Trachea: the windpipe, which may be compressed or displaced by a goitre.

Triiodothyronine: colloquially known as T_3, is one of the two thyroid hormones.

Tumour: a tumour is a lump or nodule that, in the context of this book, can be felt in the thyroid gland. It may be benign or cancerous.

Ultrasound scan: this is a technique for determining the structure of an organ. It is useful for investigating a goitre and may reveal a nodule or nodules that cannot be felt by your doctor, and show whether the lump is solid or cystic (filled with fluid).

Units of measurement: most drugs are measured in milligram (mg) quantities. One milligram is equivalent to 1000 micrograms (mcg or µg). If you are prescribed 0.1 mg thyroxine, this is equivalent to 100 mcg or µg of thyroxine, and 0.05 mg thyroxine is equivalent to 50 mcg or µg thyroxine.

For the measurement of hormones different units may be used in different parts of the world. In some areas, such as the United States, traditional or conventional units of weight per unit of plasma are used; in others the International System of Units (SI) is used, for example in the United Kingdom and elsewhere in Europe, whereby the molecular concentration, rather than the weight, of the hormone per unit of plasma is given. Plasma is blood from which the cellular elements (the red and white corpuscles) have been removed. For example, the total thyroxine level may be shown in the United States by weight as micrograms (μg) of thyroxine per unit of plasma (usually per 100 ml or dL), the normal reference range being about 4.0–11.0 μg/dL. In some other countries the total thyroxine level in the plasma may be expressed as the number of molecules of thyroxine per unit volume (usually one litre or L) of plasma, for example 140 nanamoles (nmol) per litre (L) of plasma, the reference range being about 58–154 nmol/L.

In the case of free thyroxine the concentration as reported in the traditional system is normally 0.7–1.7 nanagrams per 100 ml (ng/dL) plasma and in the SI systems 9–25 picomoles per litre (pmol/L) plasma.

The total thyroxine level expressed in traditional units (ng/dL) can be converted to SI units (nmol/L) by multiplying by 12.87.

Viral thyroiditis: this is the same as subacute viral thyroiditis or de Quervain's disease.

Vitamin B$_{12}$: failure to absorb this vitamin causes Addisonian anaemia. This is an autoimmune disorder caused by the destruction of certain cells in the stomach wall that secrete the intrinsic factor that facilitates the absorption of vitamin B$_{12}$. Addisonian anaemia may occur as an accompaniment of thyroid autoimmune disease.

Vitiligo: this is a skin condition characterized by patches of depigmentation surrounded by a thin rim of hyperpigmentation. It is an autoimmune disorder that may act as a marker for other autoimmune disorders.

Von Basedow's disease: this is the same as Graves' disease and named after the German doctor who also described the condition. It is the name used on the continent of Europe for diffuse toxic goitre.

Glossary of drugs

Throughout the text the common (generic) name has been used for each drug mentioned, names likely to be familiar to doctors world-wide. Doctors sometimes prescribe drugs of a particular proprietary brand and this may confuse the patient who may not know the chemical content of the proprietary tablet or its generic name.

Below is a short glossary of the drugs most often used in the treatment of patients with thyroid disorders. In each instance the drug is identified first by its common name and then by its official name as it appears in the pharmacopoeia. This is followed by a list of proprietary names, a list that cannot be all-inclusive because different brand names are used in different countries and in different marketing areas throughout the world. Finally, a brief indication is given of the purpose for which the drug is usually used.

Thyroxine (T_4)

Official names: levothyroxine sodium, L-thyroxine sodium, levothyroxinum natricum, thyroxine sodium.

Proprietary names: Cytolen, Eferox, Elthyrone, Eltroxin, Euthyrox, Eutirox, Levaxin, Levoid, Levothroid, Levothyroid, Levothyrox, Levotirox, Oroxine, Percutacrine Thyroxinique, Ro-Thyroxine, Synthroid, Thevier, Thyrax, Thyroxinal.

Use: As replacement therapy in deficiency of thyroid hormone; for treatment of goitre and of thyroid cancer.

Triiodothyronine (T_3)

Official names: liothyronine sodium, liothyroninum natricum, L-tri-iodothyronine, sodium liothyronine, triiodothyronine sodium.

Proprietary names: Cynomel, Cytomel, J-Tiron, Linomel, Ro-Thyronine, Tertroxin, Thybon, Thyrotardin, Tironina, Ti-Tre, Trithyrone.

Use: As replacement therapy in deficiency of thyroid hormones.

Mixtures of thyroxine and triiodothyronine

Official names: none.

Proprietary names: Liotrix (available in a range of strengths containing T_4 and T_3 in a 4:1 ratio), Euthyroid, Thyrolar.

Use: As replacement therapy in deficiency of thyroid hormones but without any proven advantage over thyroxine alone.

Thyroid extract

Official names: dry thyroid, Getrocknete Schilddrüse, thyroid extract, thyreoidin, thyroidea, thyroideum sicca, tiroide secca.

Proprietary names: Armour Thyroid, S-P-T, Thyranon, Thyrar, Thyreoid, Thyrobiline, Thyrocrine, Thyroidine, Tiroides.

Use: As replacement therapy in deficiency of thyroid hormone; largely superceded by thyroxine because thyroid extract is not a pure substance.

Carbimazole

Official names: carbimazole, carbimazolum.

Proprietary names: Basolest, Carbazole, Carbotiroid, Neo-carbimazole, Neo-Mercazol, Neo-Mercazole, Neo-Morphazole, Neo-Thyreostat, Neo-Tireol, Neo-Tomizol.

Use: For control or treatment of thyroid overactivity.

Methimazole

Official names: mercazolylum, thiamazole, tiamazol.
Proprietary names: Antitiroide GW, Danantizol, Favistan, Mercaptol, Metazolo, Strumazol, Tapazole, Thacapzol, Thycapazol, Tirodril, Tomizol.
Use: For control or treatment of thyroid overactivity.

Propylthiouracil

Official names: propylthiouracilum.
Proprietary names: Propycil, Propyl-Thyracil, Thyreostat II, Tiotil.
Use: For control or treatment of thyroid overactivity.

Propranolol

Official name: propranolol hydrochloride.
Proprietary names: Angilol, Apsolol, Avlocardyl, Bedranol, Beprane, Berkolol, Beta-Neg, Bétaryl, Beta-Tablinen, Beta-Temelits, Blocadryl, Cardinol, Cardispare, Caridolol, Deralin, Detensol, Dociton, Efektotol, Elbrol, Euprovasin, Frekven, Herzul, Inderal, Inderalici, Indobloc, Kemi, Noloten, Novopranol, Oposim, Pranolol, Prano-Puren, Prolol, Pronovan, Propobbloc, Propalong, Propayerst, Propranur, Pur-Bloka, Pylapron, Rexigen, Sagittol, Sumial, Tensiflex, Tesnol, Tonum.
Use: To slow the heart rate and reduce other symptoms of thyroid overactivity.

Glossary of Patient-Support Organizations

Australia	Thyroid Foundation of Australia PO Box 186 Westmead 2145
Canada	Thyroid Foundation of Canada (TFC) La Foundation Canadienne de la Thyroide Suite C, 1040 Gardiners Road Kingston, Ontario K7P 1R7
Denmark	Thyreoidea Landsforeningen Abakkevej 55, st. tv 2720 Vanlose
Germany	Schilddrüsen Liga Deutschland e.V. (SLD) Postfach 800740 D 65907 Frankfurt
Italy	Associazione Italiana Basedowiani e Tiroidei (AIBAT) c/o Centro Minerva Via Mazzini 6 43100 Parma
The Netherlands	Schildklierstichting Nederland (SSN) Postbus 138 1620 AC Hoorn

Glossary of patient-support groups

Sweden	Vastsvenska patient-Föreningen för Sköldkörtel Sjoka (VPFS) Mejerivalen 8 43936 Onsala
United Kingdom	British Thyroid Foundation PO Box HP22, Leeds LS6 3RT
	Thyroid Eye Disease (TED) 34 Fore Street Chudleigh Devon TQ13 0HX
USA	National Graves' Disease Foundation 2 Tsitsi Court Brevard, NC 28712
	Thyroid Foundation of America Ruth Sleeper Hall 350 Parkman Street Boston, MA 02114–2698

Index

Index